I0649542

EXERCISE
in the
CLINICAL
MANAGEMENT
of
DIABETES

Barbara N. Campaigne, PhD
American College of Sports Medicine, Indianapolis, IN

Richard M. Lampman, PhD
Catherine McAuley Health System, Ann Arbor, MI

Human Kinetics

Library of Congress Cataloging-in-Publication Data

Campaigne, Barbara N., 1951-
    Exercise in the clinical management of diabetes / Barbara N.
Campaigne and Richard M. Lampman.
        p.   cm.
    Includes index.
    ISBN 0-87322-634-8
    1. Diabetes--Exercise therapy.   I. Lampman, Richard M., 1943-
II. Title.
    RC661.E94C35   1994
    616.4'62062--dc20   93-43321
                                                                               CIP

ISBN: 0-87322-634-8   #29386651

Developmental Editor: Mary E. Fowler; Assistant Editors: Anna Curry, Ed Giles,
Pam Johnson, Lisa Sotirelis; Copyeditor: Ginger Rodriquez; Proofreader: Steve
Wrone; Indexer: Theresa J. Schaefer; Production Director: Ernie Noa; Typesetting
and Pagination: Angela K. Snyder; Text Designer: Keith Blomberg; Cover Designer:
Jack Davis; Cover Graphic: Eli Lilly and Company; Interior Illustrations: Studio
2 D; Printer: Braun-Brumfield

Photo on page 1 provided courtesy of Eli Lilly and Company.

Much of this text was written while Dr. Campaigne was working at Children's Hospital
Medical Center in Cincinnati, Ohio.

Printed in the United States of America

10   9   8   7   6   5   4   3   2   1

Human Kinetics
P.O. Box 5076, Champaign, IL 61825-5076
1-800-747-4457

Canada: Human Kinetics, Box 24040,
Windsor, ON N8Y 4Y9
1-800-465-7301 (in Canada only)

Europe: Human Kinetics
P.O. Box IW14, Leeds LS16 6TR, England
0532-781708

Australia: Human Kinetics, P.O. Box 80,
Kingswood 5062, South Australia
618-374-0433

New Zealand: Human Kinetics, P.O. Box 105-231,
Auckland 1
(09) 309-2259

To Mom and Pop, whose love, support, and belief in me has made all the difference; and to God, my foundation. This book is dedicated in part to all the individuals who have, had, or will have diabetes. May it in some way enlighten and lighten them along their way. And to Marilyn Martens, co-founder of Human Kinetics, whom I never knew, but felt a deep compassion towards because of the bond of diabetes.
BC

To my children, Brian, Collin, and Carly, the joy of my life, for their love, understanding, support, and forbearance.
RL

Contents

Preface   vii

Acknowledgments   ix

Chapter 1   Diabetes Mellitus: Etiology and Pathology   1

Type I Diabetes 1
Type II Diabetes 4
Normal Insulin Secretion 7
Abnormal Insulin Secretion 8
Hepatic and Peripheral Insulin Resistance 10
Abnormal Hepatic Glucose Production and Diminished Peripheral
    Uptake 11
Lipid and Lipoprotein Abnormalities 12
Complications of Diabetes 14
Treatment of Type I and Type II Diabetes 16
Normal Response to Exercise: Cardiovascular and Metabolic Changes
    and Adaptations 17
Exercise and Chronic Disease States 19
Exercise in the Clinical Management of Diabetes 20

Chapter 2   Acute Exercises in Type I Diabetes   35

Blood Glucose in Diabetes 35
Glucose Regulation 37
Insulin Sensitivity 42
Exercise 44

Chapter 3   Physical Training in Type I Diabetes   61

Blood Glucose Control 61
Insulin Sensitivity 67
Skeletal Muscle Metabolism 72
Serum Lipids and Lipoproteins 75
Epidemiological Evidence 77

Chapter 4   Metabolic and Physiologic Responses to Acute Exercise in Type II Diabetes   85

Substrate Utilization in People Without Diabetes 86
Type II Diabetes 92
Acute Exercise and Glycemic Control 93
Diabetes and Cardiovascular Response to Acute Exercise 101

Chapter 5   Physical Training in the Management of Type II Diabetes   115

Physical Training in People Without Diabetes   115
Physical Training in Type II Diabetes   117

Chapter 6   The Clinical Application of Exercise in Type I Diabetes   139

Screening   140
Design and Implementation of the Exercise Program   141
Exercise and Complications of Diabetes   152
Case Studies   162

Chapter 7   The Clinical Application of Exercise in Type II Diabetes   169

Screening and Medical Evaluation   171
Potential Adverse Effects of Physical Training   172
Preexercise Training Evaluation   173
Exercise Prescription: Systematic Approach   173
Injury Prevention and Safety Considerations   178
Metabolic Control   178
Environmental Considerations, Attire, and Shoes   179
Exercise Equipment   180
Clinical Applications   180
Model Treatment Programs   180
Managing Patients With Special Needs   182
Case Studies   182

Glossary   189
Index   195
About the Authors   211

Preface

Diabetes is a unique disease affecting many organ systems. Because exercise has proven to have beneficial effects on both glucose and insulin metabolism, health professionals have begun to recommend it as a therapeutic intervention. However, because of the diversity of diabetes, the individuality of responses to exercise, and associated cardiovascular complications, no standard guidelines have been developed for the systematic use of exercise. *Exercise in the Clinical Management of Diabetes* represents a unique contribution to the field of exercise science. This book includes an extensive literature review and focuses on the metabolic environment of Type I and Type II diabetes and the effects of exercise on the disease.

We've written *Exercise in the Clinical Management of Diabetes* to establish or develop conclusions about the benefits and use of exercise to prevent, lessen, or reverse many of the metabolic abnormalities present in people with Type I and Type II diabetes mellitus. Our intent is to help you discern when exercise is appropriate and beneficial and when it is not. It is our aim to offer guidelines for applying exercise with patients in the clinical setting to prevent, delay the onset of, or treat diabetes.

This book should prove to be a valuable resource on metabolic, hormonal, and cardiovascular responses to acute and chronic exercise and training, on the particular risk associated with this clinical management technique, and on precautions to prevent undesirable events. We provide scientific and clinical information valuable for a multidisciplinary audience involved in diabetes treatment and research—exercise physiologists, nurses, health care workers, physician assistants, physiologists, diabetologists, epidemiologists, and biochemists. Professionals who work with patients in clinical settings such as cardiac rehabilitation or diabetes management programs will also find the book helpful, and it contains important information for the person with diabetes who wants to participate in recreational and competitive sports. In addition, the book is a valuable reference for researchers and students in exercise science and could serve as a supplementary text for coursework.

Many questions remain unanswered about the benefits of exercise for people with diabetes. We hope that *Exercise in the Clinical Management of Diabetes* will foster the systematic use of exercise to improve euglycemic control and prevent the manifestations of diabetes. We also hope that it will enable those of you who advise patients about exercise to promote exercise safety, optimal performance, enjoyment, and success.

The more that is known about exercise and diabetes, the more precisely we will be able to formulate recommendations and guidelines. We hope that with this book we can make a contribution to the ultimate goal of reducing the effects of diabetes and offering improved quality of life to people with the disease.

Acknowledgments

I wish to tenderly acknowledge the following individuals whose love, support, and encouragement over the years has made this book possible: Rainer Martens and Mary Fowler who helped the vision come true, Lizzie, Brian, Bruce, Julie, George, Lynn and Amy, who supported the effort patiently over the years. A special thanks for the hard work, care, and technical assistance of Margie, Sheila, Vicki, and Marilyn.

BC

Chapter 1

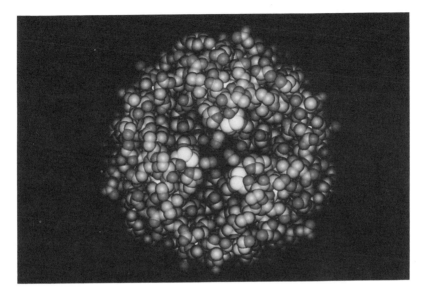

Diabetes Mellitus: Etiology and Pathology

Diabetes is commonly broken down into two types: insulin-dependent (Type I) and non-insulin-dependent (Type II). A basic understanding of the characteristics of both types is essential to determining the possible benefits and use of exercise in the prevention, reversal, and control of these two very distinct diseases. In this chapter we examine the factors, such as genetics, the environment, and demographics, that have been found to possibly contribute to the development of both types of diabetes. We also present general information about the metabolic complications associated with diabetes and set the scene for discussing how exercise can be used in the management of these conditions.

Type I Diabetes

Insulin-dependent diabetes mellitus (IDDM) or Type I diabetes, previously known as juvenile-onset diabetes, is believed to be an inherited *autoimmune* disease. Diabetic populations carry *histocompatibility antigens*

1

with a diabetes-specific genetic code. Type I diabetes occurs in 10% to 15% of diabetes cases in the Western world, but its incidence shows marked geographic differences worldwide. For example, people in Scandinavian countries are 35 times more likely to develop diabetes than people in Japan (LaPorte et al., 1985) (Figure 1.1). A positive relationship between a given country's incidence of Type I diabetes and its distance from the equator has been reported (R = 0.76) (LaPorte et al.).

Etiology of Type I Diabetes

Type I diabetes appears heterogeneous in terms of genetic, autoimmune, and environmental factors that bring about the disease (Rimoin & Rotter, 1981; Rotter & Rimoin, 1981). Type I diabetes shows a strong correlation with inherited histocompatibility antigen types (chromosome 6 encoded), and with various degrees of cell-mediated and serologic autoimmunity. The immune response is thought to be triggered by an environmental condition such as a viral infection or chemical agent—it has been associated with viral inflammation at or near the onset of the disease (Fajans,

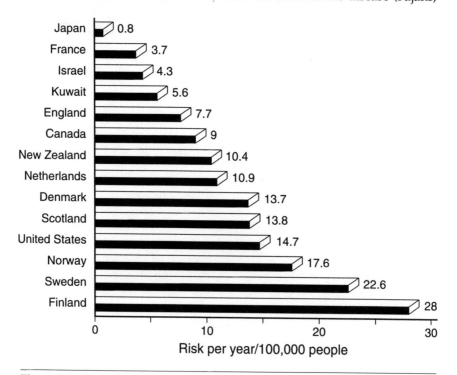

Figure 1.1   The relative risk per year of developing insulin-dependent diabetes mellitus by country.
Reprinted with permission from *Diabetes Care*, **8**, 1985, p. 103. Copyright © 1985 by American Diabetes Association, Inc.

1989). Most important, Type I diabetes is characterized by an eventual absence of endogenous insulin production, as measured by circulating *C-peptide* levels. Insulin resistance (when normal insulin levels fail to produce a normal response) is also present, but its pathogenesis is not well understood (DeFronzo, Hendler, & Simonson, 1982).

Type I diabetes occurs commonly in childhood and adolescence. However, it can be recognized and become symptomatic at any age. In the early stages of the disease, usually within the first year, the pancreas has some residual beta cell function. During this time of remission patients may withdraw from insulin completely and later maintain near-normal glucose levels with one insulin injection daily. This *"honeymoon" phase* usually lasts anywhere from a few weeks to a few years. Following this phase, insulin administration is essential to prevent ketosis, coma, and death. The individual with Type I diabetes experiences wide swings in blood glucose levels and usually requires multiple daily insulin injections.

A second type of insulin-dependent diabetes (Type IB) occurs less commonly—it is present in about 10% of Type I cases. Primary autoimmunity is thought to be the cause of this disease, in which patients have associated autoimmune endocrine disease, such as Grave's disease, Addison's disease, Hashimoto's thyroiditis, and primary gonadal failure, along with associated nonendocrine autoimmune disease, such as connective tissue disease, pernicious anemia, myasthenia gravis, and celiac disease. Type 1B occurs more commonly in females than males, and the onset of symptoms does not take place until individuals are 30 to 50 years of age.

Prognosis in Type I Diabetes

Prior to the discovery of insulin, the Type I patient usually died from *ketoacidosis* within 2 years of the onset of diabetes. After the discovery of insulin around 1921, the problem of premature death was thought to be solved. However, in the 1940s and 1950s doctors found that patients who had been managed on insulin therapy for 20 to 30 years had developed the previously mentioned specific complications of the disease (retinopathy, nephropathy, neuropathy). The discovery of these "silent" complications led to the use of daily multiple insulin injections in treating Type I patients with the hope that carefully evaluated and broadly applied attempts at tighter glucose control would provide a brighter outlook for individuals with Type I diabetes.

Glycemic Control

Within the past 20 years *hemoglobin* A_{1c} (HbA_{1c}) or glycosylated hemoglobin, a unique hemoglobin molecule, has been characterized (Bunn, Haney, Kamin, Gabbay, & Gallop, 1976). The hemoglobin is chemically bound to a glucose molecule and constitutes about 5% of the hemoglobin in a normal red blood cell. In diabetics it may be 2 to 4 times higher than normal, because, in general, the higher the circulating glucose concentration, the greater the amount of HbA_{1c} formed. This *glycosylation* results in a small decrease in the ability of the red cell to transport oxygen. Recent evidence shows that high concentrations of blood glucose lead to glycosylation of other proteins, including serum albumin, red cell membrane proteins, myelin, and others, and of tissues as well (Brownlee, Vlassara, & Cerami, 1984; Monnier & Cerami, 1983). Glycosylated hemoglobin has a life of around 3 to 4 months, or the life of a red blood cell. This makes it a good method for assessing long-term blood glucose control in both Type I and Type II patients.

Type II Diabetes

Type II diabetes mellitus is commonly called non-insulin-dependent diabetes mellitus (NIDDM). It was known previously as maturity-onset or adult-onset diabetes. Of individuals with diabetes, 90% have Type II diabetes. Diabetes affects more than 6.5 million Americans or 3 percent of the U.S. population. There are probably an equal number of people with undiagnosed cases. In Western countries overall, it affects 3% to 7% of adults (World Health Organization Study Group, 1985). Diabetes mellitus and impaired glucose tolerance are highly prevalent among older adults. Data from the National Health and Nutrition Examination Survey (NHANES) collected from 1976 to 1980 indicate that nearly 10% of Americans 65 to 74 years old had been previously diagnosed with diabetes mellitus. An equal number were found to have undiagnosed NIDDM, and an additional 25% of this elderly population had impaired glucose tolerance to an oral glucose load (Harris, Hadden, Knowler, & Bennett, 1987). The prevalence of NIDDM increases with age, with an annual incidence of 0.5% to 1% over age 65 compared with less than 0.2% at ages 24 to 44. The overall prevalence of NIDDM increased approximately 5% annually during the same period, with the majority of the increase in the elderly (Herman et al., 1984). Type II diabetes is frequently seen in many other parts of the world (Bennett, 1990) and has a high prevalence in populations of the Pacific Islands (Polynesians and Micronesians), Australian Aborigines and migrant Asian-Indians. NIDDM is more common in Native Americans (for example, an estimated 20% to 25% of Pima Indians have the disease) than among U.S. Caucasians (Wingard, Sinsheimer, Barrett-Connor, & McPhillips, 1990; Zimmet & Whitehouse, 1979). Type II diabetes is also more prevalent among African-Americans and Hispanics (The Carter Center of Emory Univeristy, 1985). The pathogenesis of NIDDM remains unknown (Leahy & Boyd, 1993; Pfeiffer & Dolderer, 1987), but it is believed to be a heterogeneous disorder with a strong genetic factor (Fajans, Cloutier, & Crowther, 1978). A major abnormal characteristic of NIDDM is insulin resistance (Reaven, 1983; Reaven, 1988). Table 1.1 shows major characteristics of Type I and Type II diabetes.

Etiology of Type II Diabetes

Environmental factors play a role in the development of NIDDM because the prevalence rate increases with obesity and aging. Approximately 80 percent of individuals with NIDDM are obese. Furthermore, obesity not only plays a role in inducing Type II diabetes, but it can also worsen glucose tolerance. Obese individuals are often hypertensive, and hypertension has been associated with hyperinsulinemia (Fournier, Gadia, Kubrusly, Skyler, & Sosenko, 1986). Recent evidence suggests a close association between insulin resistance, glucose intolerance, and hyperinsulinemia in patients with hypertension (Swislocki, Hoffman, & Reaven, 1989). The close association among NIDDM, obesity, dyslipidemia, and hypertension (Reaven, 1991) has important implications for increasing the risk of developing arteriosclerosis (Pollare, Lithell, & Berne, 1990; Robertson & Strong, 1968). Atherosclerotic macrovascular disease of both coronary and peripheral arteries is the primary cause of mortality in patients with NIDDM. It is postulated that hyperinsulinemia accelerates the development of arteriosclerosis (Stolar, 1988). An individual with NIDDM, therefore, is usually obese, is over the age of 30 years, and is often without classic symptoms of diabetes mellitus until later years (National Diabetes Data Group, 1979).

NIDDM is characterized by diminished insulin secretion relative to serum glucose levels and peripheral insulin resistance, both of which can be exacerbated by chronic hyperglycemia and improved by euglycemia. Individuals with the disease have abnormalities in both hepatic glucose production and glucose uptake in the peripheral tissues (DeFronzo, Simonson, & Ferrannini, 1982; Kolterman et al., 1981). In contrast to Type I diabetes, circulating pancreatic islet cell antibodies are not present, beta-cell destruction does not occur (Gepts, 1983), and pancreatic beta cell insulin secretion remains relatively intact (DeFronzo, Simonson, & Ferrannini, 1982).

NIDDM is characterized by three major metabolic abnormalities:

- Impairment in pancreatic beta cell insulin secretion in response to a glucose stimulus (DeFronzo, Ferrannini, & Koivisto, 1983; Halter, Graf, & Porte, 1979)
- A reduced sensitivity to the action of insulin in major organ systems such as muscle, liver, and adipose tissue (DeFronzo, Deibert, Hendler, Felig, & Soman, 1979; DeFronzo et al., 1983; Olefsky, Kolterman, & Scarlett, 1982)
- Excessive hepatic glucose production in the basal state (Gerich, 1984; Revers, Fink, Griffin, Olefsky, & Kolterman, 1984)

Table 1.1   The Major Characteristics of Type I and Type II Diabetes Mellitus

Factor	Type I	Type II
Age of onset	Usually early, but may occur at any age	Usually over age 30, but may occur at any age
Type of onset	Usually abrupt	Insidious
Genetic susceptibility	HLA-related DR3, DR4, and others	Frequent genetic background, not HLA-related
Environmental factors	Virus, toxins, autoimmune stimulation	Obesity, nutrition
Islet-cell antibody	Present at onset	Not observed
Endogenous insulin	Minimal or absent	Stimulated response is either adequate but delayed secretion or reduced but not absent; insulin resistance present
Nutritional status	Thin, catabolic state	Obese or may be normal
Symptoms	Thirst, polyuria, polyphagia, fatigue	Mild or frequently none
Ketosis	Prone; at onset or during insulin deficiency	Resistant; except during infection or stress
Control of diabetes	Often difficult with wide glucose fluctuation	Variable; helped by dietary adherence, weight loss, and exercise
Dietary management	Essential	Essential; may suffice for glycemic control
Insulin	Required for all	Required for 20% to 30%
Oral hypoglycemics	Not effective	Effective
Vascular and neurologic complications	Seen in majority after 5 or more years of diabetes	Frequent

From "Diabetes Mellitus: Definition, Classification, and Diagnosis" by C.R. Shuman. In *Diabetes Mellitus* (9th ed.) by J.A. Galloway, J.H. Potvin, and C.R. Shuman (Eds.), 1988, Indianapolis, IN: Lilly Research Laboratories. Copyright 1988 by Eli Lilly and Company. Adapted by permission.

It remains unclear whether these conditions occur simultaneously, or if one precedes the other.

Normal Insulin Secretion

In an individual who is not diabetic, two distinct phases of insulin secretion occur in response to a glucose stimulus (see Figure 1.2) (Ward, Beard, & Porte, 1986). The early-phase response appears within 3 min following a glucose stimulus and lasts for about 10 min. This early insulin secretion represents readily available insulin stored in the pancreatic beta cells (Ward et al., 1986). In the later phase, newly synthesized insulin is secreted in relation to the level and rate of increase of the blood glucose concentration (Ward et al., 1986).

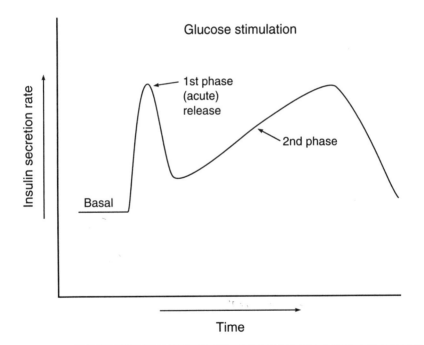

Figure 1.2   The biphasic insulin response to a constant glucose stimulus showing a theoretical response to a square-wave (constant) change in glucose concentration. The peak of the first phase in humans is between 3 and 5 min and lasts 10 min. The second phase begins at 2 min but is not evident until 10 min have passed. It continues to increase slowly for at least 60 min or until the stimulus stops.

Reprinted with permission from *Diabetes Care*, **7**, 1984, p. 492. Copyright © 1984 by American Diabetes Association, Inc.

Abnormal Insulin Secretion

Fasting plasma insulin levels can be low, normal, or elevated in subjects with NIDDM (DeFronzo, Hendler, et al., 1982). If individuals are matched for fasting glucose levels and degree of obesity, however, those with Type II diabetes show reduced basal insulin concentrations (Halter et al., 1979; Ward, Beard, Halter, Pfeiffer, & Porte, 1984).

Insulin secretion abnormalities can be demonstrated in the subject with NIDDM using a standard oral glucose tolerance test. The decrease or absence of the early phase of insulin secretion is characteristic of the individual with NIDDM (Pfeiffer, Halter, & Porte, 1987). In response to an oral glucose challenge, glucose intolerant individuals with a fasting plasma glucose level less than 115 mg/dl usually have normal or slightly elevated insulin secretion. When basal insulin levels are normal or elevated relative to slightly elevated glucose levels, basal insulin secretion rates increase in response to reduced insulin sensitivity and hyperglycemia. Individuals with elevated glucose levels (over 115 mg/dl) usually show a diminished early-phase insulin secretion response to an oral glucose challenge. Pyke (1986) has suggested that this sluggish insulin release may be associated with genetic factors because a high concordance rate of Type II diabetes has been found in identical twins. Whether the early phase of insulin secretion is necessary for priming target tissue and to what extent it contributes to postprandial hyperglycemia in NIDDM are unknown.

The late insulin-release phase during an oral glucose challenge may be normal in an individual with moderate fasting hyperglycemia (140 to 180 mg/dl). Although these individuals may have late-phase insulin release similar to that of individuals who are not diabetic, their insulin secretion is inadequate because its action is reduced (insulin resistance). On the other hand, the late phase of insulin secretion may be elevated in a nondiabetic person with insulin resistance. For individuals with severe hyperglycemia (plasma glucose levels greater than 180 to 200 mg/dl), insulin secretion is usually nonexistent.

With time, defects both in insulin secretion and insulin resistance become markedly worse, and moderate to severe fasting hyperglycemia (plasma glucose greater than 180 to 200 mg/dl) occurs. Although total insulin secretion may be subnormal, normal, or elevated, it is insufficient to normalize hyperglycemia (Fraze et al., 1985). An abnormally high basal insulin secretion rate in response to hyperglycemia is found in subjects with NIDDM, but this resulting hyperinsulinemia is attenuated over that noted in healthy individuals with similar plasma-glucose levels (Polonsky et al., 1986). If the disease progresses to marked fasting hyperglycemia (glucose levels greater than 250 to 300 mg/dl), beta cell function is severely impaired and the fasting insulin level is diminished (Polonsky et al., 1986).

In general, normal plasma glucose levels are associated with normal pancreatic beta cell function, whereas in hyperglycemia insulin secretion is below normal or lacking. Because of impaired insulin secretion in the early phase, hepatic glucose production is uncontrolled as glucose enters the system via the gastrointestinal tract. The net effect is marked hyperglycemia that is not suppressed until many hours later in response to delayed hyperinsulinemia. As the diabetes worsens, this late phase of insulin secretion decreases, allowing for more prolonged periods of hyperglycemia.

The pulsating characteristics of insulin are abnormal in obese individuals as well. Insulin resistance is compensated for by augmented insulin secretion in the obese, nondiabetic person, but not to the level that is sufficient to maintain normal glycemia. The major difference between individuals who are obese and nondiabetic and nonobese individuals with diabetes is that the people who have diabetes are unable to release sufficient amounts of insulin to overcome their insulin resistance (DeFronzo et al., 1983). With obesity, hyperinsulinemia is probably due to both increased pancreatic beta cell insulin secretion and diminished hepatic clearance of insulin (Polonsky et al., 1986). As illustrated in Figure 1.3, thin and obese patients with NIDDM have a blunted increase and delayed peak in serum insulin concentration relative to healthy individuals (Bagdade, Bierman, & Port, 1967).

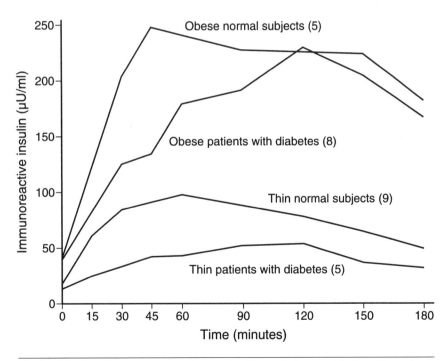

Figure 1.3   Insulin response to glucose in thin and obese subjects with and without NIDDM.

Reproduced from the *Journal of Clinical Investigation*, 1967, **46**, pp. 1549-1557 by copyright permission of the American Society for Clinical Investigation.

Hepatic and Peripheral Insulin Resistance

Insulin resistance is a major factor contributing to hyperglycemia in the individual with NIDDM. It is characterized by a diminished response to the action of insulin in hepatic and other peripheral tissues (Olefsky, 1985). DeFronzo et al. (1979), utilizing the *euglycemic* clamp technique to determine peripheral insulin resistance, showed less binding of insulin to adipocytes in subjects with NIDDM. If the individual is also obese, a reduced number of binding sites and a decrease in insulin receptor kinase activity are factors contributing to insulin resistance (see Figure 1.4) (Caro et al., 1987). Insulin receptor *downregulation* from prolonged compensatory hyperinsulinemia may also be a factor in decreased insulin binding. In this condition, binding affinity to receptors remains normal, but there are a decreased number of insulin receptors (Kolterman et al., 1981). In addition to a decrease in the number, the structure of the insulin receptor, its function, or both are altered (Taylor et al., 1990). Studies have shown that both obese and nonobese individuals with NIDDM have combined receptor and postreceptor defects (Kashiwagi et al., 1983; Kolterman et al., 1981), but coupling between insulin receptor binding and insulin effector unit activation remains normal (Kolterman, Insel, Saekow, & Olefsky, 1980). A proposed schema for the resulting insulin resistance of NIDDM is shown in Figure 1.5.

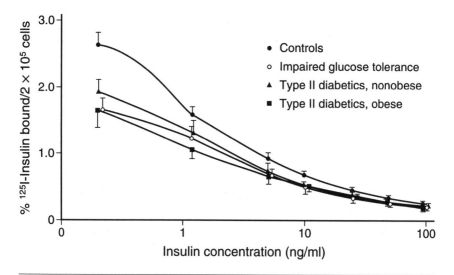

Figure 1.4   Insulin binding by isolated adipocytes. All data are corrected for nonspecific binding and represent the mean ± standard error of the percentage of ^{125}I insulin specifically bound per 2×10^5 cells.
Reproduced from the *Journal of Clinical Investigation*, 1981, **68**, p. 961 by copyright permission of the American Society for Clinical Investigation.

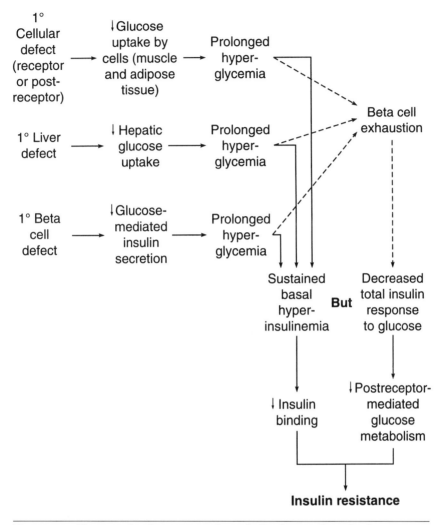

Figure 1.5   The postulated sequence of metabolic abnormalities leading to insulin resistance in NIDDM.

From "New Cocnepts in the Pathogenesis and Treatment of Non-Insulin-Dependent Diabetes Mellitus" by R.A. DeFronzo, E. Ferrannini, and V. Koivisto, 1983, *American Journal of Medicine*, **74**(Suppl. 1a), pp. 52-81. Copyright 1983 by The American Journal of Medicine. Reprinted by permission.

Abnormal Hepatic Glucose Production and Diminished Peripheral Uptake

Another disorder present in subjects with NIDDM is hepatic overproduction of glucose resulting in progressive hyperglycemia and continued reduced insulin sensitivity (DeFronzo, Simonson, et al., 1982), thought to be secondary to hepatic insulin resistance. Support for this abnormality is the close relationship between hepatic glucose production and fasting hyperglycemia in subjects with NIDDM (DeFronzo et al., 1979; Revers et al., 1984). In this situation, hepatic insulin resistance is present because fasting hyperinsulinemia usually occurs yet excess hepatic glucose production exists (DeFronzo et al., 1983). Accelerated hepatic glucose output is the greatest contributor to elevated basal glucose levels observed in NIDDM, and augmented gluconeogenesis rather than glycogenolysis plays the predominant role in increased hepatic glucose output (Consoli, Nuijhan, Capani, & Gerich, 1989). A diminished insulin supression of free fatty acids (FFA) provides a ready fuel source for gluconeogenesis via FFA oxidation. This enhances hepatic glucose production and consequently elevates plasma glucose levels (Rifkin, 1991). The pathogenesis of postprandial hyperglycemia in NIDDM is due primarily to diminished suppression of endogenous hepatic glucose and, to a lesser extent, decreased hepatic glucose sequestration (Mitrakou et al., 1990).

The inability of insulin to suppress hepatic glucose production and the inability of insulin to stimulate glucose utilization in target tissue are both contributing factors to the hyperglycemia found in NIDDM (Gerich, 1984). Healthy, normal-weight individuals dispose of glucose at a rate of 6.4 mg/kg/min, whereas those with NIDDM display a glucose uptake rate of only 4.6 mg/kg/min (DeFronzo et al., 1979). Golay, DeFronzo, Thorin, Jequier, and Felber (1988), utilizing the euglycemic and hyperinsulinemic clamp techniques, demonstrated that impairment in total body glucose uptake resulted primarily from a defect in nonoxidative glucose disposal. This diminished response was greatest in obese diabetic individuals followed by obese nondiabetics and, finally, normal-weight diabetics as compared with nonobese, nondiabetic controls. Of interest also was the finding that total glucose oxidation was lower for both diabetic groups, but not for the obese nondiabetic individuals as compared with the normal-weight control group. The reduced postabsorptive systemic glucose clearance in NIDDM does not appear to be solely related to skeletal muscle, because less than 10% of impaired glucose clearance is due to muscle in the rested state (Gerich et al., 1990).

Lipid and Lipoprotein Abnormalities

Lipid abnormalities are present in both Type I and Type II diabetes (see Table 1.2). Just as abnormalities in insulin and carbohydrate metabolism are major defects in subjects with diabetes, abnormalities in lipid and lipoprotein metabolism are also a prominent characteristic of NIDDM. These lipid abnormalities may be related to poor glycemic control and hyperinsulinemia. Evidence suggests a close link between chronic hyperinsulinemia and the development of atherosclerosis (Stanby, 1968; Swislocki et al., 1989). A close negative relationship has been reported between

Table 1.2   Common Lipid Abnormalities of Diabetes

Lipid	Type I	Type II
HDL-CHOL	Normal	Low
LDL-CHOL	High	High
Triglycerides	High	High
Total cholesterol	High	High

plasma insulin levels and high-density lipoprotein (HDL) cholesterol levels, and a positive association has been found between insulin and triglyceride levels. Both correlations implicate insulin resistance as an etiology for these coronary artery disease risk factors (Laws, King, Haskell, & Reaven, 1991). The close associations among hyperinsulinemia, hyperglycemia, and dislipidemia are important considerations when implementing therapeutic approaches for those with diabetes because of their high prevalence of cardiovascular disease.

An abnormally high triglyceride level is a common feature of Type II diabetes (Albrink, 1974). Triglyceride levels are elevated due to an increase in plasma very low density lipoprotein (VLDL) triglyceride synthesis and secretion (Greenfield, Kolterman, Olefsky, & Reaven, 1980) and to a decreased peripheral clearance of triglycerides (Reaven, 1987). Because VLDL carries approximately 20% cholesterol, total cholesterol levels may be elevated in subjects with NIDDM. The other major lipid abnormality in individuals with NIDDM is reduced HDL cholesterol concentrations (Greenfield, Doberne, Rosenthal, Vreman, & Reaven, 1982; Nikkila, 1981). Low levels of HDL cholesterol are closely associated with elevated levels of triglycerides. The reason for reduced HDL cholesterol levels is unknown, but it may relate to a higher catabolic rate of apoprotein A-1/HDL (Golay et al., 1987).

These two lipoprotein abnormalities result in altered lipid metabolism in hyperglycemic states (Reaven, 1987). Work reported by Greenfield et al. (1982) suggests a relationship between abnormalities in lipoprotein metabolism and glycemic control in individuals with NIDDM. Insulin resistance associated with NIDDM may alter hepatic VLDL triglyceride synthesis and secretion because hyperinsulinemia and hypertriglyceridemia are closely linked (Tobey, Greenfield, Kraemer, & Reaven, 1981). The postulated sequence of these abnormalities is shown in Figure 1.6. Because postprandial lipoprotein metabolism abnormalities occur in those with fasting hypertriglyceridemia and NIDDM, they also may potentiate the already atherogenic basal lipid and lipoprotein profile (Lewis et al., 1991).

Lipid profiles associated with Type I diabetes are characterized primarily by elevated total cholesterol and normal or slightly elevated HDL

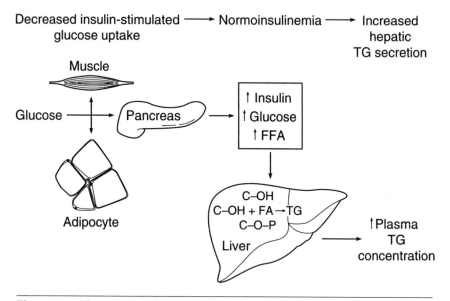

Figure 1.6   The postulated sequence of events leading to very low density lipoprotein–triglyceride secretion and hypertriglyceridemia in NIDDM.

cholesterol levels. Those in poor glycemic control display hypertriglyceridemia secondary to chylomicronemia and possible reduced HDL cholesterol levels (Bagdade, Porte, & Bierman, 1967). Mann et al. (1978) reported improvements in lipid profiles, a decrease in total cholesterol and total triglycerides, and an increase in HDL-cholesterol after a period of improved glycemic control in Type I patients. As in Type II diabetes, these abnormalities may be related to glycemic control.

Complications of Diabetes

Both Type I and Type II diabetes are greatly affected by associated complications of the disease. Several million people are diagnosed with Type I diabetes in the Western world each year, and as many as 50% of them will develop severe complications. All individuals with diabetes are at a high risk of developing *microvascular*, as well as *macrovascular*, complications (Table 1.3).

Thus, diabetes is associated with accelerated atherosclerosis development, and people with the disease are predisposed to specific microvascular complications, including *retinopathy, nephropathy,* and *neuropathy.* Diabetes increases the risk of heart disease twofold to threefold (Garcia, McNamara, Gordon, & Kannel, 1974). Peripheral vascular occlusive arterial disease and other vascular problems, particularly of the feet, are elevated 50 times. The risk of cerebral stroke doubles.

Table 1.3   The Complications of Diabetes

Acute	Chronic
Ketoacidosis (Type I)	Neuropathy peripheral autonomic
Nonketotic Hyperosmolar Coma (Type I)	Nephropathy
Lactic Acidosis (Rare—Type I)	Retinopathy background preproliferative proliferative
Hypoglycemia	Skin and connective tissue disorders Cardiovascular disease Lipid abnormalities Hypertension

An estimated 2 to 3 million individuals in the United States have Type I diabetes. Of these, close to 50% will die as a result of renal disease, as many as 20% will become blind, and virtually all will have premature atherosclerosis. The life expectancy of someone with diabetes is reduced to two thirds that of the nondiabetic individual. Because of its early onset, in most cases diabetes can lead to psychosocial maladjustment problems, especially for young patients whose activities may be restricted and who may be "sheltered" from many normal experiences. However, in most cases there is no reason for them not to live relatively normal active lives.

Type II diabetes, which is common throughout the world, may be even more prevalent because it is frequently undiagnosed until advanced symptoms or complications occur (Crofford, 1975; Harris et al., 1987). Diabetes has a major impact on health care costs—along with the disease itself is the higher risk for multiple medical problems that influence many organ systems and lead to high rates of morbidity and mortality (Marks & Krall, 1971). Of these, the most noted are atherosclerotic cardiovascular disorders (Ruderman & Haudenschild, 1984) leading to myocardial infarctions, stroke, blindness, kidney failure, and peripheral gangrene (Beach, Brunzell, Conquest, & Strandness, 1979; Beach & Strandness, 1980; Kannel & McGee, 1979; Williamson, Kilo, & Crespin, 1977).

Although a detailed understanding of the many metabolic disorders of diabetes mellitus is lacking (Colwell, Lopes-Virella, & Halushka, 1981; Keen & Jarrett, 1982), various macrovascular, microvascular, and neuropathic diseases associated with diabetes mellitus suggest that abnormalities exist in carbohydrate, insulin, fat, and protein metabolism (Jarrett, Keen, & Chakrabarti, 1982; Reaven & Steiner, 1981; Ruderman &

Haudenschild, 1984). The pathogenesis of hypertension has been closely linked to hyperinsulinemia, possibly due to increased renal tubular reabsorption of sodium, increased sympathetic activity, or both (Reaven & Hoffman, 1987). Others have noted that essential hypertension emerges as a prominent risk factor along with abnormalities of carbohydrate, insulin, and lipid metabolism in those with insulin resistance associated with Type II diabetes (Ferrannini et al., 1987; Krotkiewski et al., 1979; Modan et al., 1985; Pollare et al., 1990; Reaven & Hoffman, 1987). The individual with NIDDM is at high risk for developing severe arteriosclerosis because of many associated factors, including insulin resistance, hyperinsulinemia, hyperglycemia, elevated VLDL triglycerides, reduced HDL cholesterol levels, and impaired fibrinolytic activity (Juhan-Vague et al., 1989; Reaven, 1988; Reaven & Hoffman, 1987). In individuals with atherosclerosis, hyperinsulinemia and insulin resistance are more prevalent, even in the absence of impaired glucose tolerance or overt obesity (Ruderman & Haudenschild, 1984; Stout, 1985). A female with diabetes is at 20 times greater risk than a nondiabetic female for developing coronary artery disease (CAD), and a diabetic male has 2 to 3 times greater risk than a nondiabetic male (Kannel & McGee, 1979; Marks & Krall, 1971). Environmental factors such as obesity and cigarette smoking increase the risk of atherosclerotic vascular disease (Ruderman & Haudenschild, 1984). People who have adopted a Western way of life with less physical exercise reportedly are at increased risk for Type II diabetes and coronary artery disease (Fujimoto et al., 1987; Kawate, Yamkido, & Nishimoto, 1979; Lillioja & Bogardus, 1988; O'Dea, 1984; Stern, Rosenthal, Haffner, Hazuda, & Franco, 1984; Zimmet, 1988).

Treatment of Type I and Type II Diabetes

Type I diabetes is treated by administering exogeneous insulin (via single or multiple subcutaneous insulin injections or continuous subcutaneous insulin infusion using an insulin "pump") with the therapeutic aim to achieve and maintain near-normal blood glucose levels. Diet is also closely monitored to achieve this aim. For both Type I and Type II patients a low-fat, carbohydrate-controlled diet, with emphasis on complex carbohydrates and reduction of simple carbohydrates, is recommended (American Diabetes Association Clinical Practical Recommendations, 1991). Exercise should be a major part of the total clinical management (Franz, 1987; Vranic & Berger, 1979).

Exogenous insulin may be necessary for adequate glycemic control in the individual with Type II diabetes. An important characteristic of Type II diabetes is that insulin resistance and insulin secretory defects usually can be reversed with nonpharmacologic therapeutic interventions, such as diet and exercise. Weight loss helps normalize glycemic control in obese patients (Lampman & Schteingart, 1988).

Exercise training has been prescribed as an adjuvant therapy for individuals with diabetes (Heath, Gavin, et al., 1983; LeBlanc, Nadeau, Boulay, & Rosseau-Migneron, 1979; Ruderman, Granda, & Johansen, 1979). Exercise has a pronounced effect on serum glucose level (Devlin & Horton, 1989), perhaps through increased insulin binding activity of insulin receptors, enhanced cell permeability to glucose, and increased peripheral glucose uptake. Exercise training may help not only to maintain glycemic control but also to lower confounding atherosclerotic risk factors, enhance cardiovascular function, and improve muscular strength in these individuals (Ekelund et al., 1988; Lampman et al., 1985; Paffenbarger, Wing, & Hyde, 1978; Ruderman, Apelian, & Schneider, 1990; Schneider, Vitug, & Ruderman, 1986).

Normal Response to Exercise: Cardiovascular and Metabolic Changes and Adaptations

Exercise training results in a variety of physiologic, metabolic, and hormonal responses depending on the type of exercise performed; the intensity and duration of effort; and the individual's physical fitness level, age, and nutritional state. Acute metabolic and physiological responses to a single exercise session are immediate and temporary. They result in rapid metabolic, cardiovascular, neural, and hormonal responses to ensure adequate mobilization, usage, and redistribution of energy sources (see Figure 1.7) (Coggan, 1991). For example, heart rate, stroke volume, cardiac output, ventilation, and systolic blood pressure increase with increasing workloads, as performed during a progressive multistage treadmill test (Astrand & Rodahl, 1971; Maksud, Coutts, & Hamilton, 1971). Energy demands of contracting skeletal muscle increase abruptly with acute exercise (Jorfeldt & Wahren, 1970), resulting in a major shift in blood flow from inactive sites to areas of high metabolic demand (Carlsten & Grimby, 1966).

Responses to chronic exercise (exercise performed regularly) are more permanent and result in physiological and metabolic adaptations that improve functional capacity and fitness level, and enhance the body's ability to respond more efficiently to subsequent acute exercise (Lamb, 1984). For example, chronic exercise results in adaptive changes that facilitate delivery of oxygen and energy substrates to working muscle. Chronic exercise or endurance exercise training involving dynamic contractions of large muscle groups for long periods (30 minutes or more) per exercise session enhances muscular strength and simultaneously improves functioning of the cardiovascular system. Exercise training increases lipolysis in adipose tissue and the capacity of skeletal muscle to

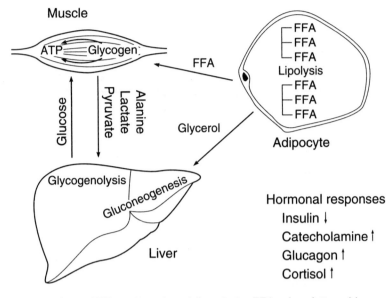

Abbreviations: ATP = adenosine triphosphate; FFA = free fatty acids.

Figure 1.7   Metabolic fuel flux and hormonal response to exercise in healthy humans.
From "Exercise in the Patient With Diabetes Mellitus" by B. Zinman. In *Diabetes Mellitus* (9th ed.) (p. 217) by J.A. Galloway, J.H. Potvin, and C.R. Shuman (Eds.), 1988, Indianapolis: Eli Lilly Research Laboratories. Copyright 1988 by Eli Lilly Research Laboratories. Reprinted by permission.

oxidize released fatty acids for energy. It improves peak oxygen consumption ($\dot{V}O_2$max), stroke volume, cardiac output, and pulmonary ventilation (Blomquist & Saltin, 1983; Huston, Puffer, & Rodney, 1985; Matoba & Gollnick, 1984; Pollock, 1973). Other adaptations associated with endurance training in previously sedentary normal individuals include reductions in total body fat, favorable changes in abnormal plasma glucose and lipid levels, and diminished plasma insulin levels and enhanced insulin action (Bjorntorp, DeJounge, Sjostrom, & Sullivan, 1976; Bjorntorp, Fahlen, & Grimby, 1972; Koivisto, Yki-Jarvinen, & DeFronzo, 1986; Lampman et al., 1977; Lampman et al., 1985; Schneider, Vitug, & Ruderman, 1986). Regular exercise may alter insulin action in tissue by increasing the number of insulin receptors (Dohm, Sinha, & Caro, 1987) and the insulin sensitive glucose transport protein (Glut 4) (Rodnick, Holloszy, Mondon, & James, 1990). In comparison, strength training alone, such as weight training, results in improved skeletal muscle strength and hypertrophy (Matoba & Gollnick, 1984), yet has less adaptive effects on substrate utilization or improved cardiovascular function.

Exercise and Chronic Disease States

Exercise testing and training have been used for many chronic disease states as an adjuvant therapy to enhance functional capacity and to reduce the risk for cardiovascular disease (see Table 1.4) and for patients with advanced coronary arteriosclerosis to improve their fitness (Greenberg, 1979; Paffenbarger & Hyde, 1984; Paffenbarger, Wing, & Hyde, 1978). Patients engaged in a cardiac rehabilitation program showed a 20% reduction in total mortality at a 3-year follow-up and a major reduction in sudden death at a 1-year follow-up (O'Connor et al., 1989). In an important epidemiological report, Helmrich, Ragland, Leung, & Paffenbarger (1991) showed that habitual physical activity was effective in preventing NIDDM, especially in those individuals at the highest risk for the disease. Exercise training, independent of its effect on plasma lipids, has been shown to markedly diminish the severity of arteriosclerosis in primates fed an atherogenic diet for 18 months (Kramsch, Aspen, Abramowitz, Kriemendahl, & Hood, 1981).

Most noteworthy is that inactivity, in itself, is an important independent risk factor for coronary artery disease (Fletcher et al., 1992; Paffenbarger & Hyde, 1984). Habitual exercise throughout life may reduce the incidence of

Table 1.4   Dimensions of Physical Activity With Proposed Mechanism of Effect, Validation Criteria, and Diseases Affected

Physical activity dimensions	Possible mechanism(s)	Possible validation criteria	Disease(s) affected
Caloric expenditure	Energy utilization	Dietary survey, doubly labeled water	CHD[a] NIDDM, obesity, cancer
Aerobic intensity	Enhanced cardiac function	Maximal oxygen uptake, historical records	CHD, NIDDM
Weight bearing	Gravitational force	Motion sensor, pedometer	Osteoporosis
Flexibility	Range of motion	Flexometer, historical records, goniometer	Disability
Muscular strength	Muscle force generation	Strength measure, historical records	Disability

[a]CHD = coronary heart disease, NIDDM = non-insulin-dependent diabetes mellitus.
From "Physical Activity Epidemiology: Concepts, Methods, and Applications to Exercise Science" by C.J. Caspersen. In *Exercise and Sport Sciences Reviews* (Vol. 17) (p. 439) by K.B. Pandolf (Ed.), 1989, Baltimore, MD: Williams and Wilkins. Copyright 1989 by Williams and Wilkins, Inc. Reprinted by permission.

coronary artery disease (Paffenbarger & Hyde, 1984; Powell, Thompson, Caspersen, & Kendrick, 1987). Favorable benefits of exercise in reducing risk factors for cardiovascular disease have been shown in other studies as well. These benefits include

- improved HDL cholesterol levels (Heath, Ehansi, Hagberg, Hinderliter, & Goldberg, 1983; Wood, Stefanick, Williams, & Haskell, 1983),
- reduced LDL cholesterol levels (Heath, Ehsani, et al., 1983; Schneider et al., 1986; Wood et al., 1983),
- reduced triglyceride levels (Lampman et al., 1977; Lampman et al., 1985), and
- reduced blood pressure in individuals with mild hypertension (Krotkiewski et al., 1979; Nelson, Jennings, Ester, and Korner, 1986; Seals & Hagberg, 1984).

Other reports have clearly shown benefits of exercise intervention following amputation (Davidoff et al., 1992; Finestone et al., 1992), and for disease states such as obesity (Lampman & Schteingart, 1988), dyslipoproteinemia (Lampman et al., 1977; Lampman et al., 1985; Lampman et al., 1987; Wood et al., 1983), rheumatoid arthritis (Harkcom, Lampman, Banwell, & Castor, 1985), chronic obstructive pulmonary disease (Belman & Mohsenifar, 1991), asthma (Cochrane & Clark, 1990), peripheral vascular disease (Hiatt, Regensteiner, Hargarten, Wolfel, & Brass, 1990), cystic fibrosis (Canny & Levison, 1987), and end-stage renal disease (Goldberg et al., 1983). Other reports indicate that chronic activity throughout life may prevent osteoporosis (Kriska et al., 1988); reduce the incidence of colon cancer (Garabrant, Peters, Mack, & Bernstein, 1984; Gerhardsson, Floderus, & Norell, 1988); and lower the prevalence of breast cancer, cancers of the reproductive system (Frisch, Wyshak, Albright, Albright, & Schiff, 1985), and cancers of nonreproductive organs in females (Frisch, Wyshak, Albright, Albright, & Schiff, 1989). In addition, exercise training results in many benefits for the elderly (Lampman & Savage, 1987; Laws & Reaven, 1990), a population prone to the development of diabetes.

Exercise in the Clinical Management of Diabetes

Diabetes is a leading cause of disability and death (Deckert, Poulsen, & Larsen, 1978), hence intervention strategies to reduce the health care costs associated with diabetes should be a major public health focus. Because exercise training has such a pronounced effect on substrate utilization, especially in lowering blood glucose concentrations, it may be of great therapeutic value for the individual with diabetes mellitus. Diabetes mellitus associated with many other physiological and metabolic abnormalities that also may benefit from exercise training, including

- reducing hyperinsulinemia,
- improving insulin sensitivity,

- reducing body fat,
- lowering blood pressure, and
- normalizing dsylipoproteinemias.

The remaining chapters will describe in detail the effects of both acute exercise and physical training in individuals with Type I and Type II diabetes, as well as the role of exercise in the clinical management of these patients, especially in respect to associated metabolic and cardiovascular diseases (Figure 1.8) (Ruderman & Schneider, 1992).

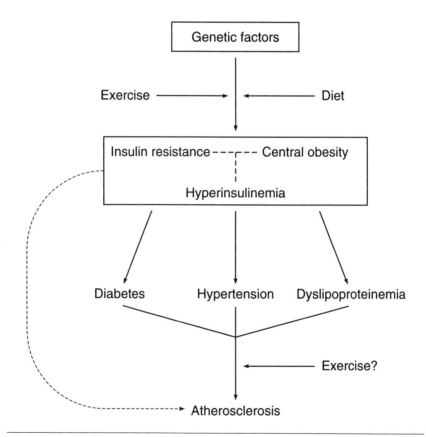

Figure 1.8   Exercise and atherosclerosis. According to this scheme, exercise and diet can modify the effect of genetic factors that predispose an individual to hyper-insulinemia, insulin resistance, and central obesity. This, in turn, will diminish the propensity of such individuals to develop Type II diabetes, hypertension, and certain dyslipoproteinemias.

Reprinted with permission from *Diabetes Care*, **15** (Suppl. 4), 1992, p. 1790. Copyright © 1992 by American Diabetes Association, Inc.

Summary

Though clearly two distinct diseases, both Type I and Type II diabetes have a hereditary component and both are influenced by environmental factors. Cultural and geographic influences play a role in the etiology of both types of diabetes. In Type I diabetes an absence of insulin production is the primary abnormality and insulin resistance is a secondary characteristic. In Type II diabetes a sequence of events stemming from insulin resistance leads to several stages of the disease involving increased insulin resistance and insulin and glucose production abnormalities.

Type I and Type II diabetes have numerous complications, many of which are common to both. Chronic cardiovascular and neurological complications may be associated with long-term elevated glucose and insulin levels, whereas acute complications are brought on by recent hyperglycemic or hypoglycemic responses. Exercise, diet, and insulin, alone or in combination, play roles in the clinical management of patients with diabetes. In subsequent chapters we will discuss current findings on acute exercise and physical training in Type I and Type II diabetes, and in the last two chapters we present specific recommendations for making exercise safe for patients and optimizing its potential use in decreasing the risk of cardiovascular disease.

References

Agner, E., Thorsteinsson, B., & Eriksen, M. (1982). Impaired glucose tolerance and diabetes mellitus in elderly subjects. *Diabetes Care*, 5, 600-604.

Albrink, M.J. (1974). Dietary and drug treatment of hyperlipidemia in diabetes. *Diabetes*, 23, 913-918.

American Diabetes Association Clinical Practice Recommendations. (1991). Nutritional recommendations and principles for individuals with diabetes mellitus: Position statement. *Diabetes Care*, 14(Suppl. 2), 20-27.

Astrand, P.O., & Rodahl, K. (1971). *Textbook of work physiology*. New York: McGraw-Hill.

Bagdade, J.D., Bierman, E.L., & Porte, D., Jr. (1967). The significance of basal insulin levels in the evaluation of the insulin response to glucose in diabetic and nondiabetic subjects. *Journal of Clinical Investigation*, 46, 1549-1557.

Bagdade, J.D., Porte, D., Jr., & Bierman, E.L. (1967). Diabetic lipemia. Form of acquired fat-induced lipemia. *New England Journal of Medicine*, 276, 427-433.

Beach, K.W., Brunzell, J.J., Conquest, L.L., & Strandness, D.E. (1979). The correlation of arteriosclerosis obliterans with lipoproteins in insulin-dependent and non-insulin dependent diabetes. *Diabetes*, 28, 836-840.

Beach, K.W., & Strandness, D.E. (1980). Atherosclerosis obliterans and associated risk factors in insulin-dependent and non-insulin dependent diabetes. *Diabetes*, **29**, 822-828.

Belman, M.J., & Mohsenifar, Z. (1991). Reductions in exercise lactic acidosis and ventilation as a result of exercise training in patients with obstructive lung disease. *American Review of Respiratory Disease*, **144**(5), 1220-1221.

Bennett, P.H. (1990). Epidemiology of diabetes mellitus. In H. Rifkin & D. Porte (Eds.), *Diabetes mellitus, theory and practice* (4th ed.) (pp. 357-377). New York: Elsevier Science.

Bjorntorp, P., DeJounge, K., Sjostrom, L., & Sullivan, L. (1976). The effect of physical training on insulin production in obesity. *Metabolism*, **19**, 631-638.

Bjorntorp, P., Fahlen, M., & Grimby, G. (1972). Carbohydrate and lipid metabolism in middle-aged physically well-trained men. *Metabolism*, **21**, 1037-1044.

Blomquist, C.G., & Saltin, B. (1983). Cardiovascular adaptations to physical training. *American Review of Physiology*, **45**, 169-189.

Brownlee, M., Vlassara, H., & Cerami, A. (1984). Nonenzymatic glycosylation and the pathogenesis of diabetic complications. *Annuals Internal Medicine*, **101**(4), 527-537.

Bunn, H.F., Haney, D.N., Kamin, S., Gabbay, K.H., & Gallop, P.M. (1976). The biosynthesis of human hemoglobin A_{1-C}. Slow glycosylation of hemoglobin in vivo. *Journal of Clinical Investigation*, **57**(6), 1652-1659.

Canny, G.J., & Levison, H. (1987). Exercise response and rehabilitation in cystic fibrosis. *Sports Medicine*, **4**(2), 143-152.

Carlsten, A., & Grimby, G. (1966). *The circulatory response to muscular exercise in man*. Springfield, IL: Charles C Thomas.

Caro, J.F., Sinha, M.K., Raju, S.M., Ittoop, O., Pories, W.J., Flickinger, E.G., Meelheim, D., & Dohm, G.L. (1987). Insulin receptor kinase in human skeletal muscle from obese subjects with and without noninsulin dependent diabetes. *Journal of Clinical Investigation*, **79**, 1330-1337.

The Carter Center of Emory University. (1985). Closing the gap: The problem of diabetes mellitus in the United States. *Diabetes Care*, **8**, 391-406.

Cochrane, L.M., & Clark, C.J. (1990). Benefits and problems of a physical training program for asthmatic patients. *Thorax*, **45**(5), 345-351.

Coggan, A.R. (1991). Plasma glucose metabolism during exercise in humans. *Sports Medicine*, **11**(2), 102-124.

Colwell, J.A., Lopes-Virella, M., & Halushka, P.V. (1981). Pathogenesis of atherosclerosis in diabetes. *Diabetes Care*, **4**, 121-133.

Consoli, A., Nuijhan, N., Capani, F., & Gerich, J. (1989). Predominant role of gluconeogenesis in increased hepatic glucose production in NIDDM. *Diabetes*, **38**, 550-557.

Crofford, O. (1975). *Report of the National Commission on diabetes*. Washington, DC: Department of Health, Education and Welfare Publications (NIH 76-1018).

Damsgaard, E.M., Faber, O.K., Froland, A., Green, A., Hauge, M., Holm, N.V., & Iversen, S. (1987). Prevalence of fasting hyperglycemia and known non-insulin-dependent diabetes mellitus classified by plasma C-peptide: Fredericia survey of subjects 60-74 yr. old. *Diabetes Care,* **10,** 26-32.

Davidoff, G.N., Lampman, R.M., Westbury, L., Deron, J., Finestone, H.M., & Islam, S. (1992). Exercise testing and training of persons with dysvascular amputation: Safety and efficacy of arm ergometry. *Archives of Physical Medicine and Rehabilitation,* **73**(4), 334-338.

Deckert, T., Poulsen, J.E., & Larsen, M. (1978). Prognosis of diabetes onset before the age of thirty-one. II. Factors influencing the prognosis. *Diabetologia,* **14,** 371-377.

DeFronzo, R., Deibert, D., Hendler, R., Felig, P., & Soman, V. (1979). Insulin sensitivity and insulin binding to monocytes in maturity onset diabetes. *Journal of Clinical Investigation,* **63,** 939-946.

DeFronzo, R., Ferrannini, E., & Koivisto, V. (1983). New concepts in the pathogenesis and treatment of noninsulin dependent diabetes mellitus. *American Journal of Medicine,* **74**(Suppl. 1A), 52-81.

DeFronzo, R.A., Hendler, R., & Simonson, D. (1982). Insulin resistance is a prominent feature of insulin-dependent diabetes. *Diabetes,* **31,** 795-801.

DeFronzo, R.A., Simonson, D., & Ferrannini, E. (1982). Hepatic and peripheral insulin resistance: A common feature of Type 2 (non-insulin-dependent) and Type 1 (insulin-dependent) diabetes mellitus. *Diabetologia,* **23,** 313-319.

Devlin, J.T., & Horton, E.S. (1989). Metabolic fuel utilization during post-exercise recovery. *American Journal of Clinical Nutrition,* **49**(5 Suppl.), 944-948.

Dohm, G.L., Sinha, M.K., & Caro, J.F. (1987). Insulin receptor binding and protein kinase activity in muscles of trained rats. *American Journal of Physiology,* **252,** E170-175.

Ekelund, L.G., Haskell, W.L., Johnson, J.L., Whaley, F.S., Criqui, M.H., & Sheps, D.S. (1988). Physical fitness as a predictor of cardiovascular mortality in asymptomatic North American men: The Lipid Research Clinic's mortality follow-up study. *New England Journal of Medicine,* **319,** 1379-1384.

Fajans, S.S. (1989). Maturity-onset diabetes of the young (MODY). *Diabetes/Metabolism Reviews,* **5**(7), 579-606.

Fajans, S.S., Cloutier, M.C., & Crowther, R.L. (1978). Clinical and etiologic heterogeneity of idiopathic diabetes mellitus. *Diabetes,* **27,** 1112-1125.

Ferrannini, E., Buzzigoli, G., Bonadonna, R., Giorico, M.A., Oleggini, M., Graziadei, L., Pedrinelli, B., Brandi, L., & Bevilacqua, S. (1987). Insulin resistance in essential hypertension. *New England Journal of Medicine,* **317,** 350-357.

Finestone, H., Lampman, R.M., Davidoff, G., Syed, S.A., Westbury, L., & Schultz, S. (1991). Arm ergometry exercise testing in the dysvascular amputee: Role of the EKG, H.R., and rate of perceived exertion in patient evaluation and exercise prescription. *Archives of Physical Medicine and Rehabilitation, 72,* 15-19.

Fletcher, G.F., Blair, S.N., Blumenthal, J., Caspersen, C., Chaitman, B., Epstein, S., Falls, H., Froelicher, E.S., Froelicher, V.F., & Pina, I.L. (1992). Statement on exercise. Benefits and recommendations for physical activity programs for all Americans. A statement for health professionals by the Committee on Exercise and Cardiac Rehabilitation of the Council on Clinical Cardiology, American Heart Association. *Circulation,* **86**(1), 340-344.

Fournier, A.M., Gadia, M.T., Kubrusly, D.B., Skyler, J.S., & Sosenko, J.M. (1986). Blood pressure, insulin, and glycemia in nondiabetic subjects. *American Journal of Medicine,* **80**(5), 861-864.

Franz, M.J. (1987). Exercise and the management of diabetes mellitus. *Journal of the American Dietetics Association,* **87**(7), 872-880.

Fraze, E., Donner, C.C., Swislock, A.L.M., Chiou, Y.A., Chen, Y.D., & Reaven, G.M. (1985). Ambient plasma–free fatty acid concentrations in noninsulin-dependent diabetes mellitus. Evidence for insulin resistance. *Journal of Clinical Endocrinology and Metabolism,* **61**, 807-811.

French, L.R., Boen, J.R., Martinez, A.M., Bushhouse, S.A., Sprafka, J.M., & Goetz, F.C. (1990). Population-based study of impaired glucose tolerance and Type II diabetes in Wadena, Minnesota. *Diabetes,* **39**, 1131-1137.

Frisch, R.E., Wyshak, G., Albright, N.L., Albright, T.E., & Schiff, I. (1985). Lower prevalence of breast cancer and cancers of the reproductive system among former college athletes compared to non-athletes. *Journal of Cancer,* **52**(6), 885-891.

Frisch, R.E., Wyshak, G., Albright, N.L., Albright, T.E., & Schiff, I. (1989). Lower prevalence of non-reproductive system cancers among female former college athletes. *Medicine and Science in Sports and Exercise,* **21**(3), 250-253.

Fujimoto, W.Y., Leonetti, D.L., Kinyoon, J.C., Shuman, W.P., Stolov, W.P., & Wahl, R.W. (1987). Prevalence of complications among second generation Japanese American men with diabetes, impaired glucose tolerance, or normal glucose tolerance. *Diabetes,* **36**, 730-739.

Garabrant, D.H., Peters, J.M., Mack, T.M., & Bernstein, L. (1984). Job activity and colon cancer risk. *American Journal of Epidemiology,* **119**, 1005-1014.

Garcia, M.J., McNamara, P.M., Gordon, T., & Kannel, W.B. (1974). Morbidity and mortality in diabetics in the Framingham population. A sixteen-year follow-up study. *Diabetes,* **23**, 105-111.

Gepts, W. (1983). Role of cellular immunity in the pathogenesis of Type I diabetes. *Current Problems of Clinical Biochemistry,* **12**, 86-107.

Gerhardsson, M., Floderus, B., & Norell, S.E. (1988). Physical activity and colon cancer risk. *Internal Journal of Epidemiology,* **17**(4), 743-746.

Gerich, J.E. (1984). Assessment of insulin resistance and its role in non-insulin dependent diabetes mellitus. *Journal of Laboratory Clinical Medicine*, **103**(4), 497-505.

Gerich, J.E., Mitrakou, A., Kelley, D., Mandarino, L., Nurjhan, N., Reilly, J., Jenssen, T., Veneman, T., & Consoli, A. (1990). Contribution of impaired muscle glucose clearance in NIDDM. *Diabetes*, **39**(2), 211-216.

Golay, A., DeFronzo, R.A., Thorin, D., Jequier, E., & Felber, J.P. (1988). Glucose disposal in obese non-diabetic and diabetic Type II patients. A study by indirect calorimetry and euglycemic insulin clamp. *Diabetes Metabolism*, **14**(4), 443-451.

Golay, A., Zech, L., Shi, M.Z. Chiou, Y.A., Reaven, G.M., & Chen, Y.D. (1987). High density lipoprotein (HDL) metabolism in non-insulin-dependent diabetes mellitus. Measurement of HDL turnover using titrated HDL. *Journal of Clinical Endocrinology and Metabolism*, **65**(3), 512-518.

Goldberg, A.P., Geltman, E.M., Hagberg, J.M., Gavin, J.R., 3rd, Delmez, J.A., Carney, R.M., Naumowicz, A., Oldfield, M.H., & Harter, H.R. (1983). Therapeutic benefits of exercise training for hemodialysis patients. *Kidney International Supplement*, **16**, S303-309.

Greenberg, M.A. (1979). The role of physical training in patients with coronary artery disease. *American Heart Journal*, **94**(4), 527-534.

Greenfield, M.S., Doberne, L., Rosenthal, M., Vreman, H.J., & Reaven, G.M. (1982). Lipid metabolism in non-insulin-dependent diabetes mellitus. Effect of Glipizide therapy. *Archives of Internal Medicine*, **142**, 1498-1500.

Greenfield, M., Kolterman, O., Olefsky, J., & Reaven, G.M. (1980). Mechanism of hypertriglyceridaemia in diabetic patients with fasting hyperglycaemia. *Diabetologia*, **18**, 441-446.

Halter, J.B., Graf, R.J., & Porte, D., Jr. (1979). Potentiation of insulin secretory responses by plasma glucose levels in man: Evidence that hyperglycemia in diabetes compensates for impaired glucose potentiation. *Journal of Clinical Endocrinology and Metabolism*, **48**(6), 946-954.

Harkcom, T.M., Lampman, R.M., Banwell, B.F., & Castor, C.W. (1985). Therapeutic value of graded aerobic exercise training in rheumatoid arthritis. *Arthritis Rheumatology*, **28**(1), 32-39.

Harris, M.E., Hadden, W.C., Knowler, W.C., & Bennett, P.H. (1987). Prevalence of diabetes and impaired glucose tolerance and plasma glucose levels in U.S. population aged 30-74 yr. *Diabetes*, **36**, 523-534.

Harris, M.I. (1989). Impaired glucose tolerance in the U.S. population. *Diabetes Care*, **12**, 464-474.

Heath, G.W., Ehansi, A.A., Hagberg, J.M., Hinderliter, J.M., & Goldberg, A.P. (1983). Exercise training improves lipoprotein lipid profiles in patients with coronary artery disease. *American Heart Journal*, **105**(6), 889-895.

Heath, G.W., Gavin, J.R., 3rd, Hinderliter, J.M., Hagberg, J.M., Bloomfield, S.A., & Holloszy, J.D. (1983). Effects of exercise and lack of exercise on glucose tolerance and insulin sensitivity. *Journal of Applied Physiology,* **55**, 512-517.

Helmrich, S.P., Ragland, D.R., Leung, R.W., & Paffenbarger, R.S., Jr. (1991). Physical activity and reduced occurrence of non-insulin-dependent diabetes mellitus. *New England Journal of Medicine,* **325**(3), 147-152.

Herman, W.H., Sinnock, P., Brenner, E., Brimberry, J.L., Langford, D., Nakashima, A., Sepe, S.J., Teutsch, S.M., & Mazze, R.S. (1984). An epidemiologic model for diabetes mellitus: Incidence, prevalence, and mortality. *Diabetes Care,* **7**, 367-371.

Hiatt, W.R., & Regensteiner, J.G. (1991). The value of exercise programs and risk factor modifications in claudicators. *Seminars in Vascular Surgery,* **4**(4), 188-194.

Hiatt, W.R., Regensteiner, J.G., Hargarten, M.E., Wolfel, E.E., & Brass, E.P. (1990). Benefit of exercise conditioning for patients with peripheral and arterial disease. *Circulation,* **81**(2), 602-609.

Huston, T.P., Puffer, J.C., & Rodney, W.M. (1985). The athletic heart syndrome. *New England Journal of Medicine,* **313**, 24-31.

Jarrett, R.J., Keen, H., & Chakrabarti, R. (1982). Diabetes, hyperglycemia and arterial disease. In H. Keen & J. Jarrett (Eds.), *Complications of Diabetes* (pp. 179-204). London: Arnold.

Jorfeldt, L., & Wahren, J. (1970). Human forearm muscle metabolism during exercise. V: Quantitative aspects of glucose uptake and production during prolonged exercise. *Scandinavian Journal of Clinical and Laboratory Investigation,* **26**, 71-81.

Juhan-Vague, I., Roul, C., Alessi, M.C., Ardissone, J.P., Herion, H., & Vague, P. (1989). Increased plasminogen activator inhibitor in non-insulin-dependent diabetic patients: Relationship with plasma insulin. *Thrombosis and Haemostatis,* **61**, 370-373.

Kannel, W.B., & McGee, D.L. (1979). Diabetes and cardiovascular disease: The Framingham study. *Journal of the American Medical Association,* **241**, 2035-2038.

Kashiwagi, A., Verso, M.A., Andrews, J., Vasquez, B., Reaven, G., & Foley, J.E. (1983). In vitro insulin resistance of human adipocytes isolated from subjects with noninsulin-dependent diabetes mellitus. *Journal of Clinical Investigation,* **72**(4), 1246-1254.

Kawate, R., Yamkido, M., & Nishimoto, Y. (1979). Diabetes mellitus and its vascular complications in Japanese migrants on the island of Hawaii. *Diabetes Care,* **2**, 161-170.

Keen, H., & Jarrett, J. (Eds.) (1982). *Complications of diabetes.* London: Arnold.

Koivisto, V.A., Yki-Jarvinen, H., & DeFronzo, R.A. (1986). Physical training and insulin sensitivity. *Diabetes Metabolic Reviews,* **37**, 924-929.

Kolterman, O.G., Gray, R.S., Griffin, J., Burstein, P., Insel, J., Scarlett, J.A., & Olefsky, J.M. (1981). Receptor and post receptor defects contribute to the insulin resistance of non-insulin-dependent diabetes mellitus. *Journal of Clinical Investigation,* **68**(4), 957-969.

Kolterman, O., Insel, J., Saekow, M., & Olefsky, J. (1980). Mechanism of insulin resistance in human obesity: Evidence for receptor and postreceptor defects. *Journal of Clinical Investigation*, **65**, 1272-1284.

Kramsch, D.M., Aspen, A.J., Abramowitz, B.M., Kriemendahl, T., & Hood, W.B., Jr. (1981). Reduction of coronary atherosclerosis by moderate conditioning exercise in monkeys on an atherogenic diet. *New England Journal of Medicine*, **305**, 1483-1489.

Kriska, A.M., Sandler, R.B., Cauley, J.A., LaPorte, R.E., Horn, D.L., & Pambianco, G. (1988). The assessment of historical physical activity and its relation to adult bone parameters. *American Journal of Epidemiology*, **127**, 1053-1063.

Krotkiewski, M., Mandrovkas, K., Sjostrom, L., Sullivan, L., Wetterquist, H., & Bjorntorp, P. (1979). Effects of long-term physical training on body fat, metabolism, and blood pressure in obesity. *Metabolism*, **28**, 650-658.

Lamb, D.R. (1984). *Physiology of exercise*. New York: MacMillan.

Lampman, R.M., Santinga, J.T., Hodge, M.F., Bassett, D.R., Block, W.D., & Flora, J.D., Jr. (1977). Comparative effect of physical training and diet in normalizing serum lipids in men with Type IV hyperlipoproteinemia. *Circulation*, **55**, 655-659.

Lampman, R.M., Santinga, J.T., Savage, P.J., Bassett, D.R., Hydrick, C.R., Flora, J.D., & Block, W.D. (1985). Effect of exercise training on glucose tolerance, in vivo insulin sensitivity, lipid and lipoprotein concentrations in middle-aged men with mild hypertriglyceridemia. *Metabolism*, **34**(3), 205-211.

Lampman, R.M., & Savage, P.J. (1987). Exercise and aging: A review of benefits and plan for action. In J.R. Sowers & J.V. Felicetta (Eds.), *The Endocrinology of Aging* (pp. 307-335). NY: Raven.

Lampman, R.M., & Schteingart, D.E. (1988). Exercise testing and prescription for the moderate and extremely obese patient. In B.A. Franklin, S. Gordon, & G.C. Timmis (Eds.), *Exercise in modern medicine: Testing and prescription in health and disease.* (pp. 156-174). Baltimore: Williams & Wilkins.

Lampman, R.M., Schteingart, D.E., Santinga, J.T., Savage, P.J., Hydrick, C.R., Bassett, D.R., & Block, W.D. (1987). The influence of physical training on glucose tolerance, insulin sensitivity, and lipid and lipoprotein concentrations in middle-aged hypertriglyceridemic, carbohydrate intolerant men. *Diabetologia*, **30**(6), 380-385.

LaPorte, R.E., Tajima, N., Akerblom, H.K., Berlin, N., Brosseau, J., Christy, M., Drash, A.L., Fishbein, H., Green, H., & Hamman, R. (1985). Geographic differences in the risk of insulin-dependent diabetes mellitus: the importance of registries. *Diabetes Care*, **8**(Suppl. 1), 101-107.

Laws, A., King, A.C., Haskell, W.L., & Reaven, G.M. (1991). Relation of fasting plasma insulin concentration to high density lipoprotein and triglyceride concentrations in men. *Arteriosclerosis and Thrombosis*, **11**(6), 1636-1642.

Laws, A., & Reaven, G.M. (1990). Effect of physical activity on age-related glucose intolerance. *Clinics in Geriatric Medicine,* **6**(4), 849-863.

Leahy, J.L., & Boyd, A.E., III. (1993). Diabetes genes in non-insulin-dependent diabetes mellitus. *The New England Journal of Medicine,* **328**(1), 56-57.

LeBlanc, J., Nadeau, A., Boulay, M., & Rousseau-Migneron, S. (1979). Effects of physical training and adiposity on glucose metabolism and 125-J insulin binding. *Journal of Applied Physiology,* **46**, 235-239.

Lewis, G.F., O'Meara, N.M., Soltys, P.A., Blockman, J.D., Iverius, P.H., Pugh, W.L., Getz, G.S., & Palonsky, K.S. (1991). Fasting hypertriglycemia in noninsulin-dependent diabetes mellitus is an important predictor of post prandial lipid and lipoprotein abnormalities. *Journal of Endocrinology and Metabolism,* **74**(4), 934-944.

Lillioja, S., & Bogardus, C. (1988). Obesity and insulin resistance: Lessons learned from the Pima Indians. *Diabetes and Metabolism Review,* **4**, 517-540.

Maksud, M.G., Coutts, K.D., & Hamilton, L.H. (1971). Time course of heart rate, ventilation and $\dot{V}O_2$ during laboratory and field exercise. *Journal of Applied Physiology,* **30**, 536-539.

Mann, J.I., Hughson, W.G., Holman, R.R., Honour, A.J., Thorogood, M., Smith, A., & Baum, J.D. (1978). Serum lipids in treated diabetic children and their families. *Clinical Endocrinology,* **27**, 27-33.

Marks, H.H., & Krall, L.P. (1971). Onset, course, prognosis and mortality in diabetes mellitus. In A. Marble, P. White, R.F. Bradley, & L. Krall (Eds.), *Joslin's Diabetes Mellitus* (pp. 209-254). Philadelphia: Lea and Febiger.

Matoba, H., & Gollnick, P.D. (1984). Response of skeletal muscles for training. *Sports Medicine,* **1**, 240-251.

Mitrakou, A., Kelley, D., Veneman, T., Jenssen, T., Pangburn, T., Reilly, J., & Gerich, J. (1990). Contribution of abnormal muscle and liver glucose metabolism to postprandial hyperglycemia in NIDDM. *Diabetes,* **39**, 1381-1390.

Modan, M., Halkin, H., Almog, S., Lusky, A., Eshkol, A., Shefi, M., Shitrit, A., & Fuchs, Z. (1985). Hyperinsulinemia: A link between hypertension, obesity and glucose intolerance. *Journal of Clinical Investigation,* **75**, 809-817.

Monnier, V.M., & Cerami, A. (1983). Detection of nonenzymatic browning products in the human lens. *Biochemistry and Biophysics Acta,* **760**(1), 97-103.

Mykkanen, L., Laakso, M., Uunsitupa, M., & Pyorala, K. (1990). Prevalence of diabetes and impaired glucose tolerance in elderly subjects and their association with obesity and family history of diabetes. *Diabetes Care,* **13**, 1099-1105.

National Diabetes Data Group. (1979). Classification and diagnosis of diabetes mellitus and other categories of glucose intolerance. *Diabetes,* **28**, 1039-1057.

Nelson, L., Jennings, G.L., Ester, M.D., & Korner, P.I. (1986). Effect of changing levels of physical activity on blood pressure and hemodynamics in essential hypertension. *Lancet, 2*, 474-476.

Nikkila, E.A. (1981). High density lipoprotein in diabetes. *Diabetes,* 30(Suppl. 2), 82-87.

O'Connor, G.T., Buring, J.E., Yusu, S., Goldhaber, S.Z., Olmstead, E.M., Paffenbarger, R.S., Jr., & Hennekens, C.H. (1989). An overview of randomized trials of rehabilitation with exercise after myocardial infarction. *Circulation, 80*(2), 234-244.

O'Dea, K. (1984). Marked improvements in carbohydrate and lipid metabolism in diabetic Australian aborigines after temporary reversion to traditional lifestyle. *Diabetes, 33*, 596-603.

Olefsky, J.M. (1985). Pathogenesis of insulin resistance and hyperglycemia in non-insulin-dependent diabetes mellitus. *American Journal of Medicine, 79*(Suppl. 3B), 1-7.

Olefsky, J.M., Kolterman, O.G., & Scarlett, J.A. (1982). Insulin action and resistance in obesity and noninsulin-dependent Type II diabetes mellitus. *American Journal of Physiology, 243*(1), E15-30.

Paffenbarger, R.S., & Hyde, R.T. (1984). Exercise in the prevention of coronary heart disease. *Preventive Medicine, 30*(1), 3-22.

Paffenbarger, R.S., Jr., Wing, A.L., & Hyde, R.T. (1978). Physical activity as an index of heart attack risk in college alumni. *American Journal of Epidemiology, 108*(3), 161-175.

Pfeiffer, E.F., & Dolderer, M. (1987). Etiopathogenesis of Type II diabetes. *Medicographia, 9*, 22-26.

Pfeiffer, M.A., Halter, J.B., & Porte, D., Jr. (1987). Insulin secretion in diabetes mellitus. *American Journal of Medicine, 70*, 579-588.

Pollare, T., Lithell, H., & Berne, C. (1990). Insulin resistance is a characteristic feature of primary hypertension independent of obesity. *Metabolism, 39*(2), 167-174.

Pollock, M.L. (1973). The quantification of endurance training programs. In J.H. Wilmore (Ed.), *Exercise and Sport Sciences Reviews* (pp. 45-71). NY: Academic.

Polonsky, K., Given, B., Hirsch, L., Beebe, C., Pugh, W., Rue, P., Galloway, J., Frank, B., & Rubenstein, A. (1986). The basal hyperinsulinemia of obesity is due to enhanced insulin secretion. *Clinical Research, 34*, 552A.

Powell, K.E., Thompson, P.D., Caspersen, C.J., & Kendrick, J.S. (1987). Physical activity and the incidence of coronary heart disease. *Annual Review of Public Health, 8*, 253-287.

Pyke, D.A. (1986). Etiology and onset of Type I diabetes mellitus. In L.P. Krall (Ed.), *Treatment of diabetes in practice* (Vol. 2, pp. 21-24). New York: Elsevier Science.

Reaven, G.M. (1983). Insulin resistance in noninsulin-dependent diabetes mellitus. Does it exist and can it be measured? *The American Journal of Medicine, 74*(Suppl. 1A), 3-17.

Reaven, G.M. (1987). Abnormal lipoprotein metabolism in non-insulin-dependent diabetes mellitus. *The American Journal of Medicine*, **83** (Suppl. 3A), 31-34.

Reaven, G.M. (1988). Role of insulin resistance in human disease. *Diabetes*, **37**, 1595-1607.

Reaven, G.M. (1991). Insulin resistance and compensatory hyperinsulinemia: Role in hypertension, dyslipidemia, and coronary heart disease. *American Heart Journal*, **121**(Pt. 2), 1283-1288.

Reaven, G.M., & Hoffman, B.B. (1987). A role for insulin in the etiology and course of hypertension? *Lancet*, **2**(8556), 435-437.

Reaven, G.M., & Steiner, G. (Eds.) (1981). Proceedings of a conference on diabetes and atherosclerosis. *Diabetes*, **30**(Suppl. 2), 1-110.

Revers, R.R., Fink, R., Griffin, J., Olefsky, J.M., & Kolterman, O.G. (1984). Influence of hyperglycemia on insulin's in vivo effects in Type II diabetes. *Journal of Clinical Investigation*, **73**, 664-672.

Rifkin, H. (1991). Current states of non-insulin-dependent diabetes mellitus (Type II): Management with glipazide. *The American Journal of Medicine*, **90**(Suppl. 6A), 3S-7S.

Rimoin, D.L., & Rotter, J.I. (1981). Genetic heterogeneity in diabetes mellitus and diabetic microangiopathy. *Hormone and Metabolic Research*, **7** (Suppl. Series), 63-72.

Robertson, W.B., & Strong, J.P. (1968). Atherosclerosis in persons with hypertension and diabetes mellitus. *Laboratory Investigation*, **18**, 538-551.

Rodnick, K.J., Holloszy, J.O., Mondon, C.E., & James, D.E. (1990). Effects of exercise training on insulin-regulatable glucose transporter protein levels in rat skeletal muscle. *Diabetes*, **39**, 1425-1429.

Rotter, J.I., & Rimoin, D.L. (1981). The genetics of the glucose intolerance disorders. *American Journal of Medicine*, **70**, 116-126.

Ruderman, N.B., Apelian, A.Z., & Schneider, S.H. (1990). Exercise in therapy and prevention of Type II diabetes. *Diabetes Care*, **13**(Suppl. 4), 1163-1168.

Ruderman, N.B., Granda, O.P., & Johansen, K. (1979). The effect of physical training on glucose tolerance and plasma lipids in maturity-onset diabetes. *Diabetes*, **28**(Suppl. 1), 89-92.

Ruderman, N.B., & Haudenschild, C. (1984). Diabetes as an atherogenic factor. *Progress in Cardiovascular Disease*, **26**(5), 373-412.

Ruderman, N.B., & Schneider, S.H. (1992). Diabetes, exercise, and atherosclerosis. *Diabetes Care*, **15**(Suppl. 4), 1787-1793.

Schneider, S.H., Vitug, A., & Ruderman, N. (1986). Atherosclerosis and physical activity. *Diabetes Metabolism Review*, **1**, 513-553.

Seals, D.R., & Hagberg, J.M. (1984). The effect of exercise training on human hypertension: A review. *Medicine and Science in Sports and Exercise*, **16**, 207-215.

Stanby, N.H. (1968). Atherosclerosis and diabetes mellitus. *Acta Pathologica, Microbiologica Et Immunologica Scandinavica*, **194** (Suppl.), 152-164.

Stern, M.R., Rosenthal, M., Haffner, S.M., Hazuda, H.P., & Franco, L.J. (1984). Sex differences in the effects of sociocultural status on diabetes and cardiovascular risk factors in Mexicans-Americans: The San Antonio Heart Study. *American Journal of Epidemiology*, **120**, 834-8351.

Stolar, M.W. (1988). Atherosclerosis in diabetes: The role of hyperinsulinemia. *Metabolism*, **37**(Suppl. 1), 1-9.

Stout, R.W. (1985). Overview of the association between insulin and atherosclerosis. *Metabolism*, **34**(Suppl. 1), 7-12.

Swislocki, A.L.M., Hoffman, B.B., & Reaven, G.M. (1989). Insulin resistance, glucose intolerance and hyperinsulinemia in patients with hypertension. *American Journal of Hypertension*, **2**, 419-423.

Taylor, S.I., Kadowaki, T., Kadowaki, H., Accili, D., Cama, A., & McKeon, C. (1990). Mutations in insulin-receptor gene in insulin-resistant patients. *Diabetes Care*, **13**, 257-279.

Tobey, T.A., Greenfield, M., Kraemer, F., & Reaven, G.M. (1981). Relationship between insulin resistance, insulin secretion, very low density lipoprotein kinetics and plasma triglyceride levels in normotriglyceridemic man. *Metabolism*, **30**, 165-171.

Tuomilehto, J., Nissinen, A., Kivela, S.L., Pekkanen, J., Kaarsalo, E., Wolf, E., Aro, A., Punsar, S., & Karvonen, M.J. (1986). Prevalence of diabetes mellitus in elderly men aged 65 to 84 years in eastern and western Finland. *Diabetologia*, **29**, 611-615.

Vranic, M., & Berger, M. (1979). Exercise and diabetes mellitus. *Diabetes*, **28**, 147-163.

Ward, W.K., Beard, J.C., Halter, J.B., Pfeiffer, M.A., & Porte, D., Jr. (1984). Pathophysiology of insulin secretion in noninsulin-dependent diabetes mellitus. *Diabetes Care*, **7**, 491-502.

Ward, W.K., Beard, J.C., & Porte, D., Jr. (1986). Clinical aspects of islet B-cell function in noninsulin-dependent diabetes mellitus. In R.A. DeFronzo (Ed.), *Diabetes/Metabolism Reviews* 2 (pp. 297-313). NY: Wiley.

West, K.M. (1983). Diabetes mellitus in nutritional support of medical practice. In H.A. Schneider, C.E. Anderson, & D.B. Coursin (Eds.), *Nutritional Support of Medical Practice* (2nd ed.) (pp. 302-319). Philadelphia: Harper & Row.

Williamson, J.R., Kilo, C., & Crespin, S.R. (1977). Vascular disease. In M.E. Levin & L.W. O'Neal (Eds.), *The Diabetic Foot* (pp. 67-90). St. Louis: Mosby.

Wingard, D.L., Sinsheimer, P., Barrett-Connor, E.L., & McPhillips, J.B. (1990). Community-based study of prevalence of NIDDM in older adults. *Diabetes Care*, **13**(Suppl. 2), 3-8.

Wood, P.D., Stefanick, M.L., Williams, P.T., & Haskell, W.L. (1983). Increased exercise levels and plasma lipoprotein concentrations—a one-year randomized controlled study in sedentary middle-aged men. *Metabolism*, **32**, 31-39.

World Health Organization Study Group. (1985). Technical report series No. 727. Geneva Switzerland: Author.

Zimmet, P.Z. (1988). Primary prevention of diabetes mellitus. *Diabetes Care, 11*, 258-262.

Zimmet, P.Z., & Whitehouse, S. (1979). The effect of age on glucose tolerance: Studies in a Micronesian population with a high prevalence of diabetes. *Diabetes, 28*, 617-623.

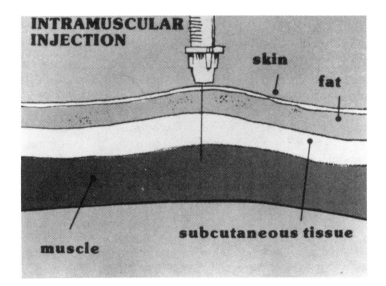

Chapter 2

Acute Exercise in Type I Diabetes

Exercise, depending on its duration and intensity, is characterized by unique endocrine and neural responses. The control of the availability and use of metabolic fuel is influenced largely by a balance of insulin, *glucagon*, and the *catecholamines* (epinephrine and norepinephrine). Other factors that may significantly influence fuel metabolism during exercise in Type I diabetes include the central nervous system (Kjaer, Secher, Bach, & Galbo, 1987), *glycemic state* (Jenkins, Furler, Chisholm, & Kraegen, 1986), and the overall metabolic profile (Cooper, Wasserman, Vranic, & Wasserman, 1986; Katz, Broberg, Sahlin, & Wahren, 1986; Wasserman & Vranic, 1985). Accordingly, this chapter will focus on the various aspects of the physiological environment of the individual with diabetes that influence the response to exercise and, conversely, how acute exercise may affect this physiological environment.

Blood Glucose in Diabetes

Because the acute response to exercise results in an increase in glucose utilization, increased glucose production is necessary to maintain near-normal blood glucose levels. As described in chapter 1, in the nondiabetic individual insulin levels fall and glucagon levels increase, as does epinephrine, to maintain near-normal blood glucose during exercise. In the person with insulin-dependent diabetes (IDDM), this becomes complicated because the *glycemic response* to exercise depends on the circulating levels of glucose and insulin, as well as the central nervous system's ability to respond appropriately, helping to elicit these hormonal responses. In the person with IDDM, exogenous insulin must be given on a regular basis to maintain near-normal glucose levels because the pancreas can no longer produce insulin. Therefore, the circulating level of insulin at the time of exercise is not physiologically controlled. The person with diabetes may also have impaired neurological function and be unable to regulate hormonal responses appropriately. This combination of factors (elevated insulin and low hormone response) results in an inability to appropriately increase glucose levels in response to the accelerated uptake of glucose that occurs during exercise.

Experimental models that mimic the metabolic environment of diabetes have been developed. When the normal response of insulin and glucose to exercise is prevented with *somatostatin* (Wolfe, Nadel, Shaw, Stephenson, & Wolfe, 1986), glucose production is hindered. In dogs, Wasserman and Abumrad (1989) found a 55% reduction in hepatic glucose output caused by attenuated *glycogenolysis*. When somatostatin was used to prevent the rise in glucagon in response to exercise, glucose production was affected by both reduced glycogenolysis and *gluconeogenesis*, resulting in a 68% reduction in glucose production. Thus, when the insulin and glucagon responses are abnormal, as is the case in diabetes, glucose levels may not be appropriately regulated. The recent work of Shilo, Sotsky, and Shamoon (1990) demonstrated that if portal insulin levels are maintained near normal during short-term mild exercise (30 min at 40% maximum capacity), glucagon secretion is necessary to maintain normal hepatic glucose release.

Glucagon release has been shown to be defective during *hypoglycemia* in patients with Type I diabetes (Cryer & Gerich, 1985; Hirsch & Shamoon, 1987). During exercise, however, glucagon secretion rates were normal in diabetic subjects, showing a direct effect of exercise on glucagon secretion (Shilo et al., 1990). Shilo et al. conclude that the hormonal regulation of glucose production during brief exercise is not dependent on decreases in portal insulin availability, as has been demonstrated during more intensive exercise, as long as an exercise-induced glucagon response can occur. However, glucagon secretion alone does not prevent hypoglycemia when portal insulin levels are increased minimally, as in Type I diabetes. This rise in glucagon and fall in insulin both affect the ability to increase glucose production, and thus it has been shown that the greatest correlate to hepatic glucose production is the ratio of glucagon to insulin (Issekutz, 1980; Wasserman, Lickley, & Vranic, 1984). It has been suggested that mobilization of hepatic glucose is controlled by the combined action of insulin and glucagon, whereas insulin and epinephrine influence exercise-induced skeletal muscle glucose uptake (Wasserman et al., 1984). Alterations in insulin, glucagon, and catecholamine levels, such as occur in diabetes, can have profound effects on glucose availability, leading to either hypo- or hyperglycemia.

The ideal to achieve in diabetes is a decreasing insulin level and an increasing glucagon level at the time of exercise, in order to promote an appropriate glucose response and maintain near-normal glucose levels. To achieve this ideal, individual patient programs must be designed as discussed later in this chapter and in chapter 6.

Glucose Regulation

Figure 2.1 illustrates the importance of insulin in influencing blood glucose levels in physically active individuals with Type I diabetes. Consider three possibilities for the patient:

- If treatment with intravenous insulin infusion generates normal portal insulin levels, glucose production will equal glucose utilization, and circulating glucose homeostasis can be maintained.
- If circulating insulin levels are low (insulin deficiency), glucose utilization may not be adequately stimulated by exercise; this in conjunction with an exercise-induced increase in hepatic glucose production may lead to hyperglycemia.
- If insulin absorption is enhanced with insulin administered subcutaneously before exercise (over insulinization), an inhibition of glucose production may result; this along with enhanced glucose utilization may lead to hypoglycemia.

Status of plasma insulin	Hepatic glucose production	Muscle glucose utilization	Blood glucose
Normal or slightly diminished	⬆	⬆	→
Markedly diminished	⬆	↑	↑
Increased	↑	⬆	↓

Figure 2.1 The influence of plasma insulin on blood glucose levels of individuals with Type I diabetes.

Glucose Uptake

Because of their complexity and invasive nature, few studies were done until recently on the influence of exercise on direct glucose uptake by skeletal muscle. Early studies by Sanders, Levinson, Abelman, and Freinkel (1964) demonstrated an increased arteriovenous (AV) difference in glucose across the leg during exercise in two subjects with diabetes. Wahren, Felig, and Hagenfeldt (1978) reported that net glucose uptake of the leg during exercise in patients with diabetes who are insulin-withdrawn and hyperglycemic is as great as in healthy controls. Glucose uptake was 13 to 18 times greater than baseline in both controls and Type I subjects after 40 min of cycling at 55% to 60% of maximal oxygen uptake. It appeared that hyperglycemic subjects favored glucose utilization by the *glycolytic* pathway, because lactate was the same as or greater than in controls. Of the total oxygen consumption by the working muscle, 25% to 30% was accounted for by glucose. Mild ketosis did not affect glucose uptake by the exercising leg.

Glucose uptake can occur in the absence of insulin (Ploug, Galbo, Vinten, Jorgensen, & Richter, 1984; Wallberg-Henriksson & Holloszy, 1984). This phenomenon has been demonstrated in vitro using epitrochlearis muscle (Baron, Brechtel, Wallace, & Edelman, 1988; Wallberg-Henriksson & Holloszy, 1985) and to a lesser extent in vivo in depancreatized dogs (Bjorkman, Miles, Wasserman, Lickley, & Vranic, 1988).

In diabetes, reduced glucose uptake occurs even under hyperglycemic conditions, which in the nondiabetic state results in an increase in glucose uptake by the mass action of glucose. This indicates that the metabolic clearance rate of glucose is reduced in diabetes. Thus, the in vitro glucose uptake response to insulin in skeletal muscle is decreased relative to controls (Klip et al., 1990; Nesher, Karl, & Kipnis, 1985; Wallberg-Henriksson & Holloszy, 1985).

Interaction Between Insulin and Exercise

The two main acute stimulators of glucose uptake into skeletal muscle are contractile activity and insulin. Although they have been well characterized (Holloszy & Narahara, 1965; Levine, Goldstein, Huddleston, & Klein, 1950; Narahara, Ozand, & Cori, 1960; Wahren, Felig, Ahlborg, & Horfeldt, 1971), the interaction between insulin and contractile activity in stimulating glucose entry into muscle is not completely understood. Studies on sartorius muscle in vitro have demonstrated that glucose transport markedly increases with electrical stimulation, even in the absence of insulin (Holloszy & Narahara, 1965). On the other hand, based on perfused hind limb preparations on rats, Berger, Hagg, and Ruderman (1975) suggest that contractile activity depends on a "permissive" amount of insulin to stimulate glucose uptake. More recent research, however, demonstrates that muscle contraction in the absence of insulin brings about glucose uptake in vitro (Richter, Ploug, & Galbo, 1985; Wallberg-Henriksson, 1986). Keep in mind that glucose uptake in vivo differs greatly from in vitro for several reasons (Klip et al., 1992). In vivo, hormonal changes occur with exercise and blood flow to muscle increases, which alters fuel availability and utilization. Sometimes changes in glycemia occur with exercise, depending on its intensity and duration, which can affect glucose uptake. The nervous system may also contribute to the increase in glucose uptake seen with exercise (Klip et al.). In addition, it has been shown that exercise and maximal insulin stimulation have additive effects on glucose transport (Wallberg-Henriksson & Holloszy, 1985). Thus, insulin stimulation and muscle contraction both increase glucose uptake. Their effects on glucose uptake may be independent and additive; further research in this area should prove fruitful.

Glucose Transport

Insulin resistance is common in Type I diabetes (Bevilacqua et al., 1985; DeFronzo, Simonson, & Ferrannini, 1982). Klip et al. (1990) reported that low basal glucose transport contributes to the defect in insulin-stimulated glucose clearance in diabetes. Alterations in glucose transport can be brought about by a defect in transporter activity or by alterations in the number of glucose transporters at the plasma membrane surface. Glucose transporters found in rat and human skeletal muscle are primarily the Glut 4 *isoform* (Birnbaum, 1989; Charron, Brosius, Alper, & Lodish, 1989; Fukumoto et al., 1989; James, Strube & Mueckler, 1989) with comparatively low levels of Glut 1 (Klip, Walker, Ransome, Schroer, & Lienhard, 1983). It appears that the Glut 4 transporter would primarily be affected by insulin and exercise because it affects glucose transport in skeletal muscle (Klip et al.).

Klip et al. (1990) showed that under *basal* conditions, the number of glucose transporters in the *intracellular membrane* (IM) is low in people with diabetes when compared with controls. They reported that insulin stimulation brings about a similar decrease in IM glucose transporters in the skeletal muscle of rats made diabetic and in control tissue. This suggests that the signal from the insulin receptor to the IM is unaltered by diabetes. The total number of transporters in skeletal muscle recruited is fewer than found in healthy controls because of the low level of glucose transporters present in diabetes. In addition, the work of Klip et al. illustrates that the increase in the number of glucose transporters recruited to the plasma membrane is lower than the number found in controls. From these findings it appears that the insulin resistance seen in conjunction with diminished glucose uptake in diabetes is caused by a decreased number of glucose transporters at the surface of the plasma membrane.

Studies of the effects of acute exercise on glucose transport have shown that muscle contraction increases the recruitment of glucose transporters to the plasma membrane (Douen, Ramlal, Klip, Young, Cartee, & Holloszy,

1989; Hirshman, Wallberg-Henriksson, Warzala, Horton, & Horton, 1988) and in a similar fashion to insulin (Klip, Ramlal, Young, & Holloszy, 1987). As mentioned, Glut 4 is recognized as the transporter isoform that is translocated to the plasma membrane with exercise. It has been suggested that two Glut 4 transporter pools exist within skeletal muscle, one induced by exercise and the other by insulin (Douen et al., 1989; Douen, Ramlal, Rastogi, et al., 1990). In addition, an increase in the activity of the glucose transporter may play a role in the increased glucose uptake seen with insulin and muscle contraction (Douen, Cartee, Ramlal, & Klip, 1990; King, Hirshman, Horton, & Horton, 1989; Nesher et al., 1985). These last two points provide fertile ground for future research. The questions to be addressed by research include these:

- Are there two glucose transporter pools within skeletal muscle? If so, what are the differential effects of insulin and exercise or muscle contraction on their recruitment?
- Do exercise or muscle contraction and insulin affect the *intrinsic* activity of the glucose transporter? If so, by what mechanism and how does the effect on the glucose transporter facilitate glucose uptake or transport?

In summary, both insulin and exercise increase glucose entry into muscle. Several findings have led to the conclusion that insulin and exercise influence glucose transport by two different mechanisms. First, the amount of time required to stimulate glucose transport occurs more rapidly with muscle contraction than with insulin (Karnielli et al., 1981). Second, unlike insulin, exercise-induced increases in glucose transport are prolonged, continuing several hours after exercise (Ivy & Holloszy, 1981; Wallberg-Henriksson & Holloszy, 1985). Third, the response to exercise and insulin may be additive (Ploug et al., 1984; Wallberg-Henriksson & Holloszy, 1984; Zorzano, Balon, Goodman & Ruderman, 1986). Last, it appears that even though the number of Glut 4 transporters in the *sarcolemma* is increased with exercise, neither insulin nor its receptor is involved (Barnard & Youngren, 1992).

Glucose Utilization and Oxidation

Because of the profound effects of insulin on glucose metabolism, glucose utilization and sources of glucose may differ in patients with Type I diabetes and healthy controls. Wahren, Hagenfeldt, and Felig (1975) have shown that during exercise glucose utilization increases similarly in Type I subjects and healthy controls. In controls, however, increased glucose utilization is attributable to an increase in glucose clearance rate, whereas in individuals with poorly controlled diabetes it appears to be primarily the result of an increase in the mass action of glucose caused by hyperglycemia, with a minor increase in glucose clearance (Bjorkman et al., 1988).

Wahren (1979) demonstrated the effects of exercise on glucose uptake by skeletal muscle and glucose production by the liver in nondiabetic healthy controls and patients with Type I diabetes. He found no significant differences between Type I subjects and healthy controls in glucose uptake by working skeletal muscle. However, he noted marked differences in hepatic glucose production by gluconeogenesis after 40 minutes of moderately heavy exercise. In individuals with diabetes, 30% of liver glucose output was accounted for by gluconeogenesis, compared to 10% for controls. Wahren et al. (1975) have shown that total hepatic glucose output rises similarly in both healthy controls and nonketotic patients with diabetes (see Figure 2.2). Among subjects with diabetes, however, the utilization of gluconeogenic *precursors* increases two to three times during short-term exercise, whereas in exercising controls the use of gluconeogenic precursors remains at basal levels. As a result, gluconeogenesis has been estimated to account for close to 30% of hepatic glucose output after moderately heavy exercise in patients withdrawn from insulin, compared with just 10% in controls.

Devlin, Scrimgeour, Brodsky, and Fuller (1994) studied the effects of moderate intensity (50% to 60% $\dot{V}O_2$max) exercise on substrate metabolism in IDDM. Subjects were studied on two occasions, during "tight" plasma glucose of 6 mM (108 mg/dl) and "loose" plasma glucose of 12 mM (216

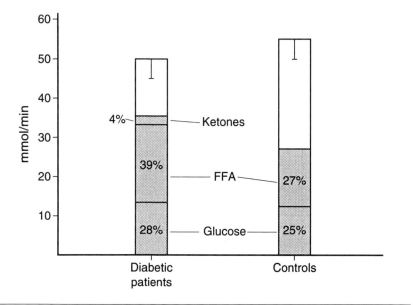

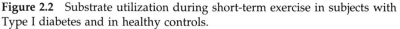

Figure 2.2 Substrate utilization during short-term exercise in subjects with Type I diabetes and in healthy controls.

Reproduced from the *Journal of Clinical Investigation*, 1975, **55**, p. 1312 by copyright permission of the American Society of Clinical Investigation.

mg/dl). On both occasions plasma glucose levels decreased during and after exercise, whereas blood ketone bodies were significantly elevated after exercise on the "loose" control day. This study clearly demonstrates that even mild insulin deficiency causing elevations in plasma glucose of 216 mg/dl may cause significant ketones in individuals with IDDM after exercise. Thus, both the glucose utilization rate and the source of glucose are affected by the state of glycemic control at the time of exercise.

Glucose oxidation appears to be altered in people with diabetes— Krzentowski et al. (1981) found that a smaller percentage of utilized glucose is fully oxidized in diabetic than nondiabetic subjects. This lower rate of glucose oxidation may be caused by impaired *pyruvate dehydrogenase* activity. An increase in *free fatty acid* utilization may in part compensate for the reduced glucose oxidation in diabetes (Wahren et al., 1975; Wahren, Sato, Ostman, Hagenfeldt, & Felig, 1984). Depending on the state of glycemic control, in Type I subjects there may also be a greater availability of *ketone* bodies for energy metabolism (Berger et al., 1977; Wahren et al., 1975; Wahren et al., 1984).

Individuals with Type I diabetes may have an altered availability of *intramuscular* substrates in response to exercise. Insulin withdrawal for 24 hr in these individuals brings about a decrease in intramuscular *glycogen* and an increase in intramuscular fat, resulting in a decreased breakdown of muscle glycogen and a rise in intramuscular fat metabolism (Standl, Lotz, Dexel, Janka, & Kolb, 1980). The individual with diabetes appears to rely more on fat metabolism than the healthy control; however, as previously mentioned, the state of insulinization prior to exercise is crucial in determining the metabolic response and substrate utilization during exercise. Thus, substrate utilization may be altered, but if insulinization is normal the metabolic response to exercise should be near normal. A summary of these findings follows:

- Hepatic gluconeogenesis elevated (after moderately heavy exercise)
- Utilization of gluconeogenic precursors elevated
- Ketone body production and utilization elevated (with mild insulin deficiency and hyperglycemia)
- Glucose oxidation reduced (incomplete)
- Free fatty acid utilization elevated
- Availability of intramuscular glycogen reduced (with insulin deficiency)
- Intramuscular fat metabolism elevated (with insulin deficiency)

Insulin Sensitivity

As previously mentioned, soon after the discovery of insulin, it was recorded that insulin requirements diminished following exercise (Lawrence, 1926).

More recent studies have described some of the possible mechanisms underlying this decreased insulin need. Increases in insulin sensitivity with exercise are well documented. Increased insulin sensitivity can last up to a day after acute exercise. Ahlborg and Felig (1982) and Devlin, Barlow, and Horton (1989) have demonstrated that nonexercised muscle releases three-carbon compounds (lactate, alanine, and pyruvate) during and immediately after exercise, which might be accounted for by glucose uptake in exercised muscle. These findings suggest that glycogenolysis of nonexercised muscle (forearm) during and after leg exercise is the source of gluconeogenic precursors for glycogen resynthesis in exercised muscle (leg). Devlin et al. (1989) found further that the forearm muscle supplying the gluconeogenic precursors was insulin resistant for 2 to 3 hr following exercise. These studies demonstrate that the increases in insulin sensitivity occurring with acute exercise are regional. Thus, increases in whole-body glucose metabolism are probably specific to local factors of previously exercised muscle (e.g., glucose transport). As Devlin (1992) suggested, the net effect of exercise on insulin sensitivity may be the sum of increases and decreases in insulin sensitivity in individual muscle groups (exercised and unexercised).

An increase in insulin sensitivity and responsiveness in muscle has been seen 3 hr after contraction, which has a large additive effect on glucose uptake (Wallberg-Henriksson, Constable, Young, & Holloszy, 1988). The increase in insulin sensitivity after muscle contraction appears to be independent of muscle glycogen levels; however, insulin responsiveness may be related to glycogen depletion (Garetto, Richter, Goodman, & Ruderman, 1984; Zarano, Balon, Goodman, & Ruderman, 1988).

Pederson, Beck-Nielsen, and Hedig (1980) reported an increase in insulin receptor number after acute exercise in well-regulated patients with Type I diabetes. This increased insulin receptor number followed both postprandial and fasting exercise. An increase in insulin binding to muscle after exercise has not been clearly demonstrated (Bonen, Tan, & Watson-Wright, 1984; Treadway, James, Burcel, & Ruderman, 1989; Zarzano, Balon, Garetto, Goodman, & Ruderman, 1985). Bonen and Tan (1989) studied the effects of a single bout of intense exercise on soleus and extensor digitorum longus (EDL) muscle in exercised and control mice. They reported that following intense exercise, insulin binding was either decreased or unchanged. Insulin-stimulated glucose uptake was increased in the EDL, but unchanged in the soleus muscle after intense exercise. However, the rate of glycogenesis was measured in both muscle groups, and glycolysis was increased in the soleus. These authors suggest a dissociation between insulin binding and glucose uptake and utilization following exercise. Although the precise mechanism behind the increased insulin sensitivity with exercise is still unknown, local effects on exercised muscle (glucose transport and utilization) appear to play a major role.

Exercise

In the Type I patient a "normal" insulin level at rest may be associated with an inappropriately elevated insulin level at the time of exercise because of the inability to decrease circulating insulin, resulting in hypoglycemia. Several findings need to be emphasized about exercise-induced hypoglycemia. Hypoglycemia may be affected by insulin injection site, elevated insulin levels brought about by exogeneous administration of insulin, and exercise intensity and duration. The acute effects of exercise on blood glucose appear to be unaffected by training. Zinman, Zuniga-Guajardo, and Kelly (1984) observed that a single exercise session resulted in a significant drop in blood glucose levels. After cycling three times a week for 45 min a session, acute exercise continued to reduce blood glucose, after both 6 weeks and 12 weeks of training. Interestingly, there was no change in insulin dose or in the number of hypoglycemic reactions during the course of the study. However, caloric intake was significantly increased on exercise days. This study supports the contention that regular exercise may require closely monitoring diet to improve metabolic control, and patients may need to increase their dietary intake to compensate for increases in activity when insulin doses are not concomitantly reduced. (For further information on physical training and glucose control, see chapter 3, pages 61-65.)

Site of Insulin Injection

It has been suggested that the site of insulin injection can affect the glycemic response to exercise in Type I patients being treated with subcutaneous insulin injections (Kawamori & Vranic, 1977; Zinman et al., 1977). However, further studies have revealed that circulating insulin levels increase to a similar extent during exercise regardless of the injection site (Kemmer et al., 1979). In this later study Kemmer et al. noted no alteration in the absorption of iodinized insulin from rest to exercise. The glycemic response to exercise was identical when insulin was injected in either the leg or the abdomen. Ferrannini, Linde, and Faber (1982), however, reported that exercise caused a twofold increase in the rate of radioactively labeled insulin disappearance from the leg in healthy volunteers during leg exercise, whereas there was no increase in the rate of disappearance from the abdominal injection site. In this study, although subcutaneous blood flow during exercise was unaltered, leg exercise was associated with a greater rise in insulin from rest to exercise than when insulin was injected in the abdomen. The glucose disappearance rate was directly related to the rise in plasma insulin concentration. Although the reduction in plasma glucose was not significantly different statistically for leg or abdomen injection, the exercise-induced reduction in glucose was 60% less after abdominal injection. This rate was not found to be statistically significant, and its clinical significance can only be speculated upon, because these subjects were healthy controls. As Berger et al. (1979) suggest, the *pharmacokinetics* of insulin may be affected by a number of factors during exercise (e.g., antibodies, type of insulin, environmental and body temperature) that need further characterization. To summarize these findings, locating the insulin injection site away from exercising muscle may be effective in preventing or delaying exercise-induced hypoglycemia in some subjects (see chapter 6).

Elevated Insulin Levels

In normal individuals insulin levels fall with exercise, as discussed in chapter 1. Because insulin levels do not decrease with exogenous administration, however, relative excess levels may occur in IDDM. Elevated circulating insulin levels lead to an inhibition of glucose production during exercise, as Kawamori and Vranic (1977) showed in depancreatized dogs and Zinman et al. (1977) showed in Type I subjects treated with intermediate-acting insulin. As discussed earlier in this chapter, when glucose production decreases simultaneously with an increase in glucose utilization by skeletal muscle, hypoglycemia will occur.

Reducing insulin dosage prior to exercise has been shown to be effective in preventing exercise-induced hypoglycemia. Thus, in patients undergoing intensive insulin therapy with normal fasting glucose levels, Schiffrin and Parikh (1985) have shown that a 30% to 50% reduction in insulin dose can prevent hypoglycemia during 45 min of *postprandial* exercise at 55% of maximal oxygen uptake. Furthermore, Kemmer and Berger (1986) have shown that individuals with diabetes can exercise for 3 hr without hypoglycemia after an 80% reduction in insulin dose, as compared with 90 min when insulin was reduced by just 50%.

Zander et al. (1983) studied the impact of heavy muscular work on substrate utilization and metabolic homeostasis in individuals with Type I diabetes. Twenty subjects with Type I diabetes were compared with 6 healthy control subjects. Subjects with diabetes were studied during hypo- and hyperinsulinemia at the start of exercise. The time of insulin injection prior to the start of exercise was used to create differences in insulin availability—hypoinsulinemia (exercise 3 hr postinjection) and hyperinsulinemia (exercise 1 hr after insulin injection). Graded exercise tests to exhaustion were used as an exercise challenge. Subjects with diabetes were found to exhibit higher heart rate responses, and their mean systolic blood pressures were higher during the last submaximal workload compared with healthy controls. In the relatively hyperinsulinemic group, exhaustive exercise resulted in significantly higher glucose and free fatty acid levels compared with people with low circulating levels of insulin. At-rest lactate concentrations were higher in the subjects with diabetes who were relatively hyperinsulinemic compared with normal controls. During exercise both groups of subjects with diabetes had significantly higher lactate levels compared with control subjects. These data reemphasize the importance of circulating levels of insulin in determining patients' substrate utilization and their response to exercise.

Treatment Modality

The mode of insulin treatment can affect the blood glucose response to exercise. The most commonly used insulin treatment regimens are continuous subcutaneous insulin infusion and multiple subcutaneous insulin injections.

Continuous Subcutaneous Insulin Infusion.   Well-controlled patients treated with continuous subcutaneous insulin infusion (CSII) can avoid exercise-induced hypoglycemia in the *postabsorptive* state (Good et al., 1983). Trovati et al. (1984) demonstrated that a group of tightly controlled patients undergoing CSII showed no differences in plasma glucose or insulin levels 2 hr after breakfast on days when subjects exercised, as compared to a control nonexercise day. These authors conclude that tightly controlled patients who are treated with CSII and perform 30 min of mild (30% to 40% $\dot{V}O_2max$) or moderate (50% to 60% $\dot{V}O_2max$) exercise, 2 to 3 hr postprandially, are not at an increased risk of developing hypoglycemia. However, it may be necessary to increase or decrease the insulin infusion in accordance with appropriate guidelines (see chapter 6, Table 6.3) to prevent hypoglycemia.

In a study, 20 patients on CSII were found to exhibit significantly lower levels of habitual physical activity than matched healthy controls and patients on multiple subcutaneous injections (Chantelau & Wirth, 1992). Physical activity levels also decreased when patients on multiple injections switched to CSII. Though the study included only a small number of patients, these findings suggest that wearing the insulin pump and catheter tubing may cause individuals treated with CSII to be less active.

Multiple Subcutaneous Injections.   Elevations in plasma glucose occur commonly after meals in individuals with diabetes. To quantify the effects of exercise on meal-induced *glycemic excursions*, Caron, Poussier, Marliss, and Zinman (1982) studied subjects undergoing standard insulin treatment by multiple subcutaneous injections (MSI) on two separate occasions, with and without 45 min of moderate exercise. For the majority of patients, exercise after breakfast prevented hyperglycemia induced by both breakfast and lunch. However, the response was variable, and exercise did not affect the glycemic response to meals in all subjects. Campaigne, Wallberg-Henriksson, and Gunnarsson (1987) studied the 12-hr plasma insulin and glucose response to moderate (60% $\dot{V}O_2max$) exercise in 10 patients and found that decreasing insulin dose or increasing dietary intake often prevented exercise-induced hypoglycemia during the 12 hr following exercise. However, as illustrated in Figure 2.3, consistent patterns of

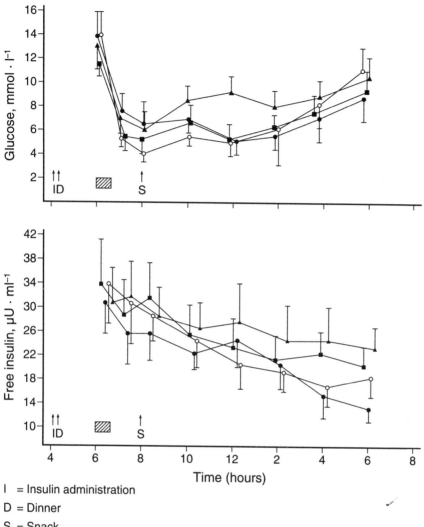

I = Insulin administration
D = Dinner
S = Snack
○ Decreased intermediate-acting insulin
● Decreased soluble insulin
▲ Increased caloric intake
■ Control
Hatched bar indicates exercise

Figure 2.3 Blood glucose (upper panel) and plasma free insulin (lower panel) concentrations in 9 insulin-dependent diabetic patients before and after 45 min of cycle exercise at 60% of maximal oxygen uptake.
From "Glucose and Insulin Responses in Relation to Insulin Dose and Caloric Intake 12 Hours After Acute Physical Exercise in Men With IDDM" by B.N. Campaigne, 1987, *Diabetes Care*, **10**(6), p. 718. Copyright 1987 by American Diabetes Association, Inc. Reprinted with permission.

plasma insulin and glucose response after exercise were observed in individual subjects after alterations in insulin or diet. Thus, specific recommendations based on individual response appear to be the best approach to preventing exercise-induced hypoglycemia in patients with diabetes.

Unlike patients receiving subcutaneous insulin injections, Type I subjects given a continuous subcutaneous insulin infusion to achieve normal arterial insulin levels have been found to have normal glucose production (Tuttle et al., 1988; Zinman et al., 1977). This phenomenon may be attributable to a relative hypoinsulinemia of the patients receiving subcutaneous insulin, caused by the inability to infuse insulin into the portal vein. Because insulin is not in the portal vein, a normal hepatic glucose production can take place. In addition, it has been shown that insulin action per se may be enhanced by exercise independent of insulin mobilization, resulting in an increased risk of hypoglycemia (Kemmer et al., 1979; Susstrunk, Morell, Ziegler, & Froesch, 1982). Thus, reducing insulin dosage prior to exercise may be appropriate in Type I individuals, especially those receiving subcutaneous insulin injections. Specific guidelines for the amount and timing of alterations in insulin dose are outlined in chapter 6.

Based on these findings, the following points may be helpful in considering insulin treatment relative to exercise:

- Inject insulin away from the exercising muscle.
- Decrease the insulin dose, especially for patients receiving insulin injections subcutaneously.
- Individualize insulin treatment.
- Consider dietary intake.

Work Intensity and Duration

To evaluate the effects of different types of exercise—short maximal exercise, 30 min of half-maximal exercise, three 10-min bouts of half-maximal exercise, and rest without exercise—Hubinger, Ridderskamp, Lehmann, and Gries (1985) studied 9 well-controlled Type I subjects on four separate occasions. Subjects were studied in the morning after they had had two thirds of their normal insulin doses to prevent hypoglycemia and had eaten a standard breakfast. Blood was analyzed for glucose, lactate, pyruvate, *free insulin*, glucagon, catecholamines, *growth hormone*, and cortisol during exercise and 60 min postexercise. Glucose was monitored for 8 hours after exercise. The findings are presented in Figures 2.4a-d. Blood glucose was unaltered by short maximal exercise. Both short-term, half-maximal and interval half-maximal exercise resulted in a decrease in blood glucose levels. The short (3-min) rest periods during the interval exercise did not alter the glucose-lowering effect or the overall *counterregulatory hormone* response when compared to continuous exercise. Maximal

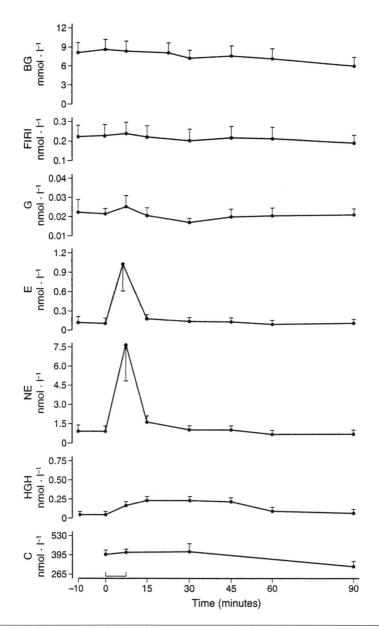

Figure 2.4a Glucose (BG), free insulin (FIRI), glucagon (G), epinephrine (E), norepinephrine (NE), growth hormone (HGH), and cortisol (C) during and after short maximal exercise.

From "Metabolic Response to Different Forms of Physical Exercise in Type I Diabetics and the Duration of the Glucose Lowering Effect" by A. Hubinger, I. Ridderskamp, E. Lehmann, and A. Gries, 1985, *European Journal of Clinical Investigation*, **15**, pp. 200-201. Copyright 1985 by Blackwell Scientific Publications Limited, Oxford, England. Reprinted by permission.

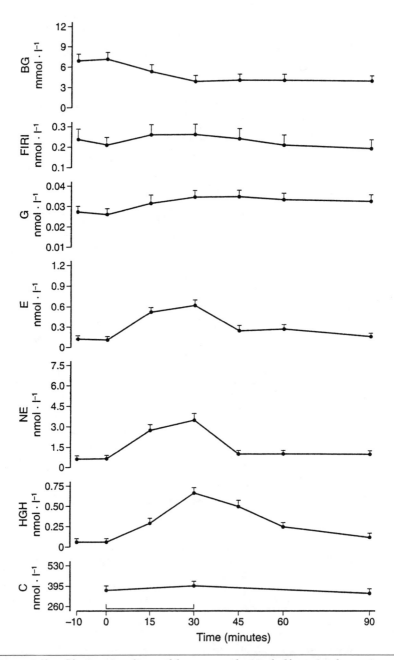

Figure 2.4b Glucose, insulin, and hormones during half-maximal exercise.
From "Metabolic Response to Different Forms of Physical Exercise in Type I Diabetics and the Duration of the Glucose Lowering Effect" by A. Hubinger, I. Ridderskamp, E. Lehmann, and A. Gries, 1985, *European Journal of Clinical Investigation*, **15**, pp. 200-201. Copyright 1985 by Blackwell Scientific Publications Limited, Oxford, England. Reprinted by permission.

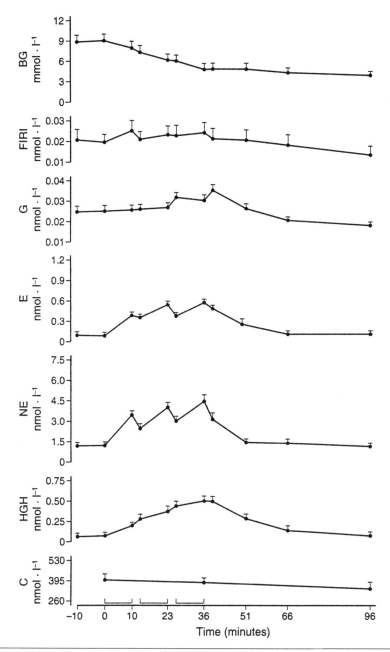

Figure 2.4c Glucose, insulin, and hormones during interval exercise.
From "Metabolic Response to Different Forms of Physical Exercise in Type I Diabetics and the Duration of the Glucose Lowering Effect" by A. Hubinger, I. Ridderskamp, E. Lehmann, and A. Gries, 1985, *European Journal of Clinical Investigation, 15*, pp. 200-201. Copyright 1985 by Blackwell Scientific Publications Limited, Oxford, England. Reprinted by permission.

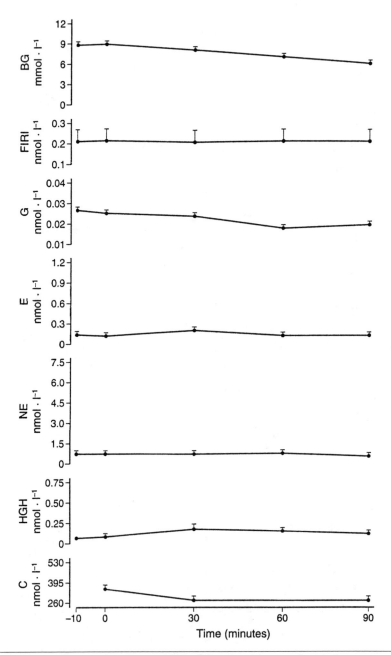

Figure 2.4d Glucose, insulin, and hormones during control period.
From "Metabolic Response to Different Forms of Physical Exercise in Type I Diabetics and the Duration of the Glucose Lowering Effect" by A. Hubinger, I. Ridderskamp, E. Lehmann, and A. Gries, 1985, *European Journal of Clinical Investigation, 15*, pp. 200-201. Copyright 1985 by Blackwell Scientific Publications Limited, Oxford, England. Reprinted by permission.

exercise produced the highest lactate and pyruvate levels, both short-term submaximal exercise sessions caused distinct increases, and the continuous and the interval exercise produced no change. Glucose values were unaffected in the afternoon following the exercise sessions. Thus, continuous or interval exercise did not elicit a long-lasting glucose-lowering effect postexercise.

These data illustrate that short-term exhaustive exercise does not appear to affect blood glucose in Type I diabetes, but both 30 min of interval exercise and 30 min of continuous exercise at a submaximal level bring about similar decreases in blood glucose. The decreases can be totally compensated for by a meal 60 min following exercise, when insulin dose has been modified by two thirds the normal amount.

Prolonged exercise resulting in hypoglycemia may be accompanied by an inappropriate counterregulatory response in some individuals with IDDM. Schneider, Vitug, Ananthakrishnan, and Khachadurian (1991) have recently demonstrated that IDDM subjects exhibited a lower norepinephrine (NE) and epinephrine (E) response to hypoglycemia after 60 min of exercise at 60% to 65% $\dot{V}O_2$max when compared with normal controls who were made similarly hypoglycemic by insulin infusion. In addition, they reported that Type I subjects had lower free fatty acid (FFA) levels than controls at the end of exercise. Glucagon and growth hormone levels did not differ between the two groups. These results suggest that hypoglycemia following prolonged moderate-intensity exercise in Type I diabetes is a result of hyperinsulinemia, combined with a low NE and E response, and a decreased availability of FFA relative to controls. It should be noted that not only the duration but also the intensity of exercise needs to be considered to determine appropriate alterations in insulin dose. High-intensity exercise appears to enhance the glucose-lowering effect of insulin compared with moderate-intensity exercise of similar duration (Hubinger et al., 1985; Zander et al., 1983).

The following points should be remembered when evaluating the effects of acute exercise on glycemic control:

- Intensity of exercise
- Duration of exercise
- Insulin injection site
- Insulin dose and mode of administration
- Glucose level prior to exercise

Summary

Individuals with diabetes must carefully consider the metabolic environment prior to the onset of exercise. In particular, it may be appropriate to adjust insulin dose and dietary intake to achieve and maintain near-normal insulin and glucose levels during and after exercise. The availability of substrates and their relative utilization and oxidation are affected by the individual's metabolic control, availability of insulin or insulin administration, and the duration and intensity of exercise. Acute exercise has a profound effect on insulin sensitivity and glucose uptake and transport. In combination with endogenously administered insulin, exercise may bring about major changes in the individual's glycemic state. The route of insulin administration, amount and timing of insulin, and the individual response to exercise warrant careful attention when considering exercise for patients with insulin-dependent diabetes.

References

Barnard, R.J., & Youngren, J.F. (1992). Regulation of glucose transport in skeletal muscle. *FASEB Journal, 6*(14), 3238-3244.

Baron, A.D., Brechtel, G., Wallace, P., & Edelman, S.V. (1988). Rates and tissue sites of non-insulin–and insulin-mediated glucose uptake in humans. *American Journal of Physiology, 255,* E769-E774.

Berger, M., Berchtold, P., Cuppers, H.J., Drost, H., Kley, H.K., Muller, W.A., Wiegelman, W., Zimmerman-Telschow, H., Gries, F.A., Kriiskemper, H.L., & Zimmerman, H. (1977). Metabolic and hormonal effects of muscular exercise in juvenile type diabetics. *Diabetologia, 13,* 355-365.

Berger, M., Hagg, S., & Ruderman, N.B. (1975). Glucose metabolism in perfused skeletal muscle. *Biochemistry Journal, 146,* 231-238.

Berger, M., Halban, B.A., Assal, J.P., Offord, R.E., Vranic, M.S., & Renold, A.E. (1979). Pharmacokinetics of subcutaneously injected tritiated insulin: Effects of exercise. *Diabetes, 28,* 53-57.

Bevilacqua, S., Barrett, E.J., Smith, D., Simonson, D.C., Olsson, M., Bratusch-Marrain, P., Ferrannini, E., & DeFronzo, R.A. (1985). Hepatic and peripheral insulin resistance following streptozotocin-induced insulin deficiency in the dog. *Metabolism, 34,* 817-825.

Birnbaum, M.M. (1989). Identification of a novel gene encoding an insulin-responsive glucose transporter protein. *Cell, 57,* 305-315.

Bjorkman, O., Miles, P., Wasserman, D.H., Lickley, L., & Vranic, M. (1988). Muscle glucose uptake during exercise in total insulin deficiency: Effect of B-Adrenergic blockade. *Journal of Clinical Investigation, 81,* 1759-1767.

Bonen, A., & Tan, M.H. (1989). Dissociation between insulin binding and glucose utilization after intense exercise in mouse skeletal muscle. *Hormone Metabolism Research, 21,* 172-178.

Bonen, A., Tan, M.H., & Watson-Wright, W.M. (1984). Effects of exercise on insulin binding and glucose metabolism in muscle. *Canadian Journal of Physiology and Pharmacology, 62,* 1500-1504.

Campaigne, B.N., Wallberg-Henriksson, H., & Gunnarsson, R. (1987). Glucose and insulin responses in relation to insulin dose and caloric intake 12h after acute physical exercise in men with IDDM. *Diabetes Care*, **10**(6), 716-721.

Caron, D., Poussier, P., Marliss, E.B., & Zinman, B. (1982). The effect of post-prandial exercise on meal-related glucose tolerance in insulin-dependent diabetic individuals. *Diabetes Care*, **5**(4), 364-369.

Cartee, G.D., Young, D.A., Sleeper, M.D., Zierath, J., Wallberg-Henriksson, H., & Holloszy, J.O. (1989). Prolonged increase in insulin-stimulated glucose transport in muscle after exercise. *American Journal of Physiology*, **256**, E494-E499.

Chantelau, E., & Wirth, R. (1992). Habitual physical activity in adult IDDM patients. A study with portable motion meters. *Diabetes Care*, **15**(4), 1727-1731.

Charron, M.J., Brosius, F.C., III, Alper, S.L., & Lodish, H.F. (1989). A novel glucose transport protein expressed predominantly in insulin-responsive tissues. *Proceedings of the National Academy of Sciences*, **86**, 2525-2539.

Cooper, D.M., Wasserman, D.H., Vranic, M., & Wasserman, K. (1986). Glucose turnover in response to exercise during high and low flow breathing in humans. *American Journal of Physiology*, **14**, E209-E214.

Cryer, P.E., & Gerich, J.E. (1985). Glucose counter-regulation, hypoglycemia and intensive insulin therapy of diabetes mellitus. *New England Journal of Medicine*, **313**, 232-241.

DeFronzo, R.A., Simonson, D., & Ferrannini, E. (1982). Hepatic and peripheral insulin resistance: A common feature of type 2 (non-insulin-dependent) and type I (insulin-dependent) diabetes mellitus. *Diabetologia*, **23**, 313-339.

Devlin, J.T. (1992). Effects of exercise on insulin sensitivity in humans. *Diabetes Care*, **15**(11), 1690-1693.

Devlin, J.T., Barlow, J., & Horton, E.S. (1989). Whole body and regional fuel metabolism during early postexercise recovery. *American Journal of Physiology*, **256**, E167-172.

Devlin, J.T., Brodsky, I., Scrimgeour, A., & Fuller, S. (1994). The mechanism of decreased protein catabolism after exercise in Type I diabetic subjects. *Diabetologia*, April.

Douen, A.G., Cartee, G., Ramlal, T., & Klip, A. (1990). Exercise modulates the insulin-induced translocation of glucose transporters in rat skeletal muscle. *Federation of European Biochemical Societies Letters*, **261**, 256-260.

Douen, A.G., Ramlal, T., Klip, A., Young, D.A., Cartee, D., & Holloszy, J.O. (1989). Exercise induced increase in glucose transporters in plasma membrane of rat skeletal muscle. *Endocrinology*, **124**, 449-454.

Douen, A.G., Ramlal, T., Rastogi, S., Bilan, P.J., Cartee, G.D., Vranic, M., Holloszy, J.O., & Klip, A. (1990). Exercise induces recruitment of the "insulin-responsive glucose transporter." [Evidence for distinct intracellular insulin- and exercise-recruitable transporter pools in skeletal muscle.] *Journal of Biological Chemistry*, **265**, 13427-13430.

Ferrannini, E., Linde, B., & Faber, O. (1982). Effects of bicycle exercise on insulin absorption and subcutaneous blood flow in the normal subject. *Clinical Physiology, 2,* 59-70.

Fukumoto, H., Kayano, T., Buse, J.B., Edwards, Y., Pilch, P.F., Bell, G.I., & Seino, S. (1989). Cloning and characterization of the major insulin-responsive glucose transporter expressed in human skeletal muscle and other insulin-responsive tissues. *Journal of Biological Chemistry, 264,* 7776-7779.

Garetto, L.P., Richter, E.A., Goodman, M.N., & Ruderman, N.B. (1984). Enhanced glucose metabolism after exercise in the rat: The two phases. *American Journal of Physiology, 246,* 471-475.

Gooch, B.R., Abumrad, N.N., Robinson, R.P., Petrik, M., Campbell, D., & Crofford, O.B. (1983). Exercise in insulin-dependent diabetes mellitus: The effect of continuous insulin infusion using the subcutaneous, intravenous and intra-peritoneal sites. *Diabetes Care, 6,* 122-182.

Goodyear, L.J., Hirshman, M.F., Smith, R.J., & Horton, E.S. (1991). Glucose transporter number, activity, and isoform content in plasma membranes of red and white skeletal muscle. *American Journal of Physiology, 261,* E556-E561.

Hirsch, B.R., & Shamoon, H. (1987). Defective epinephrine and growth hormone responses in Type I diabetes are stimulus specific. *Diabetes, 36,* 20-26.

Hirshman, M.F., Wallberg-Henriksson, H., Warzala, L.J., Horton, E.D., & Horton, E.S. (1988). Acute exercise increases the number of plasma membrane glucose transporters in rat skeletal muscle. *Federation of European Biochemical Societies Letters, 238,* 235.

Holloszy, J.O., & Narahara, H.T. (1965). Studies of tissue permeability. X. Changes in permeability to 3-methylglucose associated with contraction of isolated frog muscle. *Journal of Biological Chemistry, 240,* 2493-3500.

Hubinger, A., Ridderskamp, I., Lehmann, E., & Gries, F.A. (1985). Metabolic response to different forms of physical exercise in Type I diabetics and the duration of the glucose lowering effect. *European Journal of Clinical Investigation, 15,* 197-203.

Issekutz, R. (1980). The role of hypoinsulinemia in exercise metabolism. *Diabetes, 29,* 629-635.

James, D.E., Strube, M., & Mueckler, M. (1989). Molecular cloning and characterization of an insulin-regulatable glucose transporter. *Nature (Lond), 338,* 83-87.

Jenkins, A.B., Furler, S.M., Chisholm, D.J., & Kraegen, E.W. (1986). Regulation of hepatic glucose output during exercise by circulating glucose and insulin in humans. *American Journal of Physiology, 250,* R411-R417.

Karnielli, E., Zarnowski, M.J., Hissin, P.J., Simpson, I.A., Salans, L.B., & Cushman, S.W. (1981). Insulin-stimulated translocation of glucose transport systems in the isolated rat adipose cell. Time course, reversal, insulin concentration dependency, and relationship to glucose transport activity. *Journal of Biological Chemistry, 256*(10), 4772-4777.

Katz, A., Broberg, S., Sahlin, K., & Wahren, J. (1986). Leg glucose uptake during maximal dynamic exercise in humans. *American Journal of Physiology,* **251,** E65-E70.

Kawamori, R., & Vranic, M. (1977). Mechanism of exercise-induced hypoglycemia in depancreatized dogs maintained on long-acting insulin. *Journal of Clinical Investigation,* **59,** 331-337.

Kemmer, F.W., Berchtold, P., Berger, M., Starke, A., Cuppers, H.J., Gries, F.A., & Zimmermann, H. (1979). Exercise-induced fall of blood glucose in insulin treated diabetics unrelated to alteration of insulin mobilization. *Diabetes,* **28,** 1131-1137.

Kemmer, F.W., & Berger, M. (1986). Therapy and better quality of life: The dichotomous role of exercise in diabetes mellitus. *Diabetes/Metabolism Reviews,* **2,** 53-68.

King, P.A., Hirshman, M.F., Horton, E.D., & Horton, E.S. (1989). Glucose transport in skeletal muscle membrane vesicles from control and exercised rats. *American Journal of Physiology,* **237,** C1128-1134.

Kjaer, M., Secher, N.H., Bach, F.W., & Galbo, H. (1987). Role of motor center activity for hormonal changes and substrate mobilization in humans. *American Journal of Physiology,* **253,** R687-R695.

Klip, A., Marette, A., Dimmitrekoudis, D., Ramlal, T., Giacca, A., Shi, Z.Q., & Vranic, M. (1992). Effects of diabetes on glucoregulation: From glucose transporters to glucose metabolism in vitro. *Diabetes Care,* **15,** 1747-1766.

Klip, A., Ramlal, T., Bilan, P.J., Cartee, G.D., Gulve, E.A., & Holloszy, J.O. (1990). Recruitment of GLUT-4 glucose transporter by insulin in diabetic rat skeletal muscle. *Biochemistry and Biophysics Research Communication,* **172,** 728-736.

Klip, A., Ramlal, T., Young, D., & Holloszy, J.O. (1987). Insulin-induced translocation of glucose transporters in rat hindlimb muscles. *FEBS Letter,* **224,** 224-230.

Klip, A., Walker, D., Ransome, K.J., Schroer, D.W., & Lienhard, G.E. (1983). Identification of the glucose transporter in rat skeletal muscle. *Archives of Biochemistry and Biophysics,* **226,** 198-205.

Krzentowski, P., Pirnay, F., Pallikarakis, N., Luyckx, A.S., Lacroix, M., Mosora, F., & Lefebvre, P.J. (1981). Glucose utilization in normal and diabetic subjects. The role of insulin. *Diabetes,* **30,** 983-989.

Lawrence, R.D. (1926). The effect of exercise on insulin action in diabetes. *British Medical Journal,* **1,** 648-650.

Levine, R., Goldstein, M.S., Huddlestun, B., & Klein, S.P. (1950). Action of insulin on the permeability of cells to free hexoses, as studied by its effect on the distribution of galactose. *American Journal of Physiology,* **163,** 70-76.

Narahara, H.T., Ozand, P., & Cori, C.F. (1960). Studies of tissue permeability. VII. The effect of insulin on glucose penetration and phosphorylation in frog muscle. *The Journal of Biological Chemistry,* **235,** 3370-3378.

Nesher, R., Karl, I.E., & Kipnis, K.M. (1985). Dissociation of the effects of insulin and contraction on glucose transport in rat epitrochlearis muscle. *American Journal of Physiology, 249,* C226-232.

Pederson, O., Beck-Nielsen, H., & Hedig, L. (1980). Increased insulin receptors after exercise in patients with insulin dependent diabetes mellitus. *New England Journal of Medicine, 302,* 886-892.

Ploug, T., Galbo, H., Vinten, J., Jorgensen, M., & Richter, E. (1984). Increased muscle glucose uptake during contraction: No need for insulin. *American Journal of Physiology, 247,* E726-E731.

Ploug, T., Stallknecht, B.M., Pedersen, O., Kahn, B.B., Ohkuwa, T., Vinten, J., & Galbo, H. (1990). Effect of endurance training on glucose transport capacity and glucose transporter expression in rat skeletal muscle. *American Journal of Physiology, 259,* E778-E786.

Richter, E.A., Ploug, T., & Galbo, H. (1985). Increased muscle glucose uptake after exercise. No need for insulin during exercise. *Diabetes, 34,* 1041-1048.

Sanders, C.A., Levinson, G.E., Abelman, W.H., & Freinkel, N. (1964). Effect of exercise on peripheral utilization of glucose in man. *New England Journal of Medicine, 172,* 220-225.

Santos, R.F., Mondon, C.E., Reaven, G.M., & Azhar, S. (1989). Effects of exercise training on the relationship between insulin binding and insulin-stimulated tyrosine kinase activity in rat skeletal muscle. *Metabolism, 38,* 376-386.

Schiffrin, A., & Parikh, S. (1985). Accommodating planned exercise in Type I diabetic patients on intensive treatment. *Diabetes Care, 8,* 337-343.

Schneider, S.H., Vitug, A., Ananthakrishnan, P., & Khachadurian, A.K. (1991). Impaired adrenergic response to prolonged exercise in Type I diabetes. *Metabolism, 40,* 1219-1225.

Shilo, S., Sotsky, M., & Shamoon, H. (1990). Eyelet hormonal regulation of glucose turnover during exercise in Type I diabetes. *Journal of Clinical Endocrinology and Metabolism, 70,* 162-172.

Standl, E., Lotz, N., Dexel, T.H., Janka, H., & Kolb, H. (1980). Muscle triglycerides in diabetic subjects. *Diabetologia, 18,* 463-469.

Susstrunk, H., Morell, B., Ziegler, W.H., & Froesch, E.R. (1982). Insulin absorption from the abdomen and the thigh in healthy subjects during rest and exercise: Blood glucose, plasma insulin, growth hormone, adrenaline, and nonadrenaline levels. *Diabetologia, 22,* 171-174.

Treadway, J.L., James, D.E., Burcel, E., & Ruderman, N.B. (1989). Effect of exercise on insulin receptor binding and kinase activity in skeletal muscle. *American Journal of Physiology, 256,* E138-144.

Trovati, M., Carta, O., Cavalot, F., Vitali, S., Banaudi, C., Lucchina, P.G., Fiocchi, F., Emanuelli, G., & Lenti, G. (1984). Continuous subcutaneous insulin infusion and postprandial exercise in tightly controlled Type I (insulin dependent) diabetic patients. *Diabetes Care, 7*(4), 327-330.

Tuttle, K., Marker, J., Dalsky, G., Schwartz, N., Shah, S., Clutter, W.E., Holloszy, J.O., & Cryer, P.E. (1988). Glucagon, not insulin, may play a secondary role in defense against hypoglycemia during exercise. *American Journal of Physiology,* **17,** E713-719.

Wahren, J. (1979). Glucose turnover during exercise in healthy man and in patients with diabetes mellitus. *Diabetes,* **28**(Suppl 1), 82-88.

Wahren, J., Felig, P., Ahlborg, G., & Jorfeldt, L. (1971). Glucose metabolism during leg exercise in men. *Journal of Clinical Investigation,* **50,** 2715-2725.

Wahren, J., Felig, P., & Hagenfeldt, L. (1978). Physical exercise and fuel homeostasis in diabetes mellitus. *Diabetologia,* **14,** 213-222.

Wahren, J., Hagenfeldt, L., & Felig, P. (1975). Splanchnic and leg exchange of glucose, amino acids, and free fatty acids during exercise in diabetes mellitus. *Journal of Clinical Investigation,* **55,** 1303-1314.

Wahren, J., Sato, Y., Ostman, J., Hagenfeldt, L., & Felig, P. (1984). Turnover and splanchnic metabolism of free fatty acids and ketones in insulin-dependent diabetics during exercise. *Journal of Clinical Investigation,* **73,** 1367-1376.

Wallberg-Henriksson, H. (1986). Insulin treatment normalizes decreased glucose transport capacity in streptozotocin-diabetic rat muscle. *Acta Physiologica Scandinavica,* **128,** 647-649.

Wallberg-Henriksson, H. (1989). Acute exercise: Fuel homeostasis and glucose transport in insulin-dependent diabetes mellitus. *Medicine and Science in Sports and Exercise,* **21,** 356-361.

Wallberg-Henriksson, H., Constable, S.H., Young, D.A., & Hollozsy, J.O. (1988). Glucose transport into rat skeletal muscle: Interaction between exercise and insulin. *Journal of Applied Physiology,* **64,** 2329-2332.

Wallberg-Henriksson, H., & Holloszy, J.O. (1984). Contractile activity increases glucose uptake in muscle of severely diabetic rats. *Journal of Applied Physiology,* **57,** 1045-1049.

Wallberg-Henriksson, H., & Holloszy, J.O. (1985). Activation of glucose transport in diabetic muscle: Response to contraction and insulin. *American Journal of Physiology,* **249**(*Cellular Physiology* 18), C233-C237.

Wasserman, D.H., & Abumrad, M.N. (1989). Physiological basis for the treatment of the physically active individual with diabetes. *Sports Medicine,* **7,** 376-392.

Wasserman, D.H., Lickley, H.L.A., & Vranic, M. (1984). Interactions between glucagon and other counterregulatory hormones during normoglycemic and hypoglycemic exercise. *Journal of Clinical Investigation,* **74,** 1404-1413.

Wasserman, D.H., & Vranic, M. (1985). Interaction between insulin, glucagon, and catecholamines in the regulation of glucose production and uptake during exercise: Physiology and diabetes. In B. Saltin (Ed.), *Biochemistry of Exercise VI* (pp. 167-179). Copenhagen: International Series on Sports Sciences.

Wolfe, R.R., Nadel, E.R., Shaw, J.H.F., Stephenson, L.A., & Wolfe, M. (1986). Role of changes in insulin and glucagon in glucose homeostasis in exercise. *Journal of Clinical Investigation, 77,* 900-907.

Zander, E., Bruns, W., Wulfert, P., Besch, W., Lubs, D., Chlup, R., & Schulz, B. (1983). Muscular exercise in Type 1 diabetics. I. Different metabolic reactions during heavy muscular work independent of actual insulin availability. *Experimental Clinical Endocrinology, 82,* 78-90.

Zinman, B., Murray, F.T., Vranic, M., Albisser, A.M., Leibel, B.S., McClean, P.A., & Marliss, E.B. (1977). Glucoregulation during moderate exercise in insulin treated diabetics. *Journal of Clinical Endocrinology and Metabolism, 45,* 641-652.

Zinman, B., Zuniga-Guajardo, S., & Kelly, D. (1984). Comparison of the acute and long-term effects of exercise on glucose control in Type I diabetes. *Diabetes Care, 7,* 515-519.

Zorzano, A., Balon, T.W., Goodman, M.N., & Ruderman, N.B. (1988). Glycogen depletion and increased insulin sensitivity and responsiveness in muscle after exercise. *American Journal of Physiology, 251,* 664-669.

Chapter 3

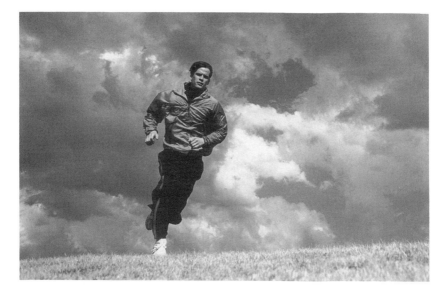

Physical Training in Type I Diabetes

Physical training is commonly defined as the performance of a given amount of exercise of a specific intensity and duration, two to three times a week over a period of weeks. The human body adapts to repeated exercise sessions. These adaptations include increased oxygen-carrying capacity, increased insulin sensitivity, improved blood lipid profiles, increased lean body mass, decreased body fatness, increased oxidative enzyme activity, and decreased resting heart rate, among others. This chapter will describe and discuss physiological changes that occur with physical training in patients with Type I diabetes.

Blood Glucose Control

That exercise lowers blood glucose was noted as early as 600 B.C. (Sushruta, 1938). Although regular exercise has been recommended for many years as an adjunct therapy for patients with Type I diabetes, its potential long-term effects for lowering blood glucose have been studied only recently.

Children/Adolescents

A summary of the effects of exercise training on glycemic control in children and adolescents is presented in Table 3.1. Changes in blood glucose control were not found after 5 months of training in adolescent males and 2 months of training in adolescent females (Larsson, Persson, Sterky, & Thoren, 1964a; Larsson, Sterky, Ekengren, & Moller, 1962). Other studies of children and adolescents have shown conflicting findings (Campaigne, Gilliam, Spencer, Lampman, & Schork, 1984; Dahl-Jorgensen, Meen, Hanssen, & Genaes, 1980; Landt, Campaigne, James, & Sperling, 1985; Rowland, Swadba, Biggs, Burke, & Ritter, 1985; Stratton, Wilson, Endres, & Goldstein, 1987). Since these studies, the availability of routine measurement of glycosylated hemoglobin has enabled studying the effects of exercise on long-term blood glucose control without daily multiple blood sampling. Glycosylated hemoglobin (HbA_1 or HbA_{1c}) is a measure of long-term blood glucose control (Compagnucci et al., 1981) because it reflects the exposure of the hemoglobin molecule to glucose over the life of a red blood cell, or approximately 3 months. HbA_{1c} is a more specific form of HbA_1. Levels of HbA_{1c} are usually 2%-3% lower than HbA_1. Dahl-Jorgensen et al. (1980) and Campaigne et al. (1984) found significant decreases in HbA_1 after physical training in children. These two studies were comparable in that both groups of children had diabetes of about 5 years duration and their initial HbA_1 levels categorized them in poor control of blood glucose (HbA_1: 13% to 15%). In contrast to these findings, however, Rowland et al. (1985) and Landt et al. (1985) found no change in blood glucose control in children and adolescents after physical training. The patients in their studies, however, were older and in better control of blood glucose before physical training began (HbA_1: 10% to 12%).

Thus, physical training in young children with short duration diabetes apparently might improve blood glucose control when initial levels of HbA_1 are high. Changes in fitness, as determined by maximal oxygen consumption ($\dot{V}O_2max$), appear to be independent of changes in HbA_1 in these patients because an increase in $\dot{V}O_2max$ was achieved in most of these studies (Landt et al., 1985; Rowland et al., 1985).

Adults

Table 3.2 summarizes the results of exercise training studies in adults. Costill et al. (1979) evaluated the effects of 10 weeks of endurance running in a group of 12 patients with Type I diabetes. These patients were compared with a group of matched healthy controls who also trained. Aerobic capacity increased significantly and to a similar extent in both groups after physical training. In the diabetic group, fasting blood glucose concentrations decreased after the training period. Muscle enzyme activities and lipid metabolism were also studied (see pages 72 and 75).

Table 3.1 Effects of Exercise on Glycemic Control in Children and Adolescents with Type I Diabetes

Author	# Patients	Control subjects	Exercise program	Glycemic control	Effect
Larsson et al., 1964	6 adolescents (6 M)	6 boys Nondiabetic	Gymnastics 5 months 1 hr, 1 × week	Glycosuria	NO
Dahl-Jorgensen et al., 1980	14 children*	8 children	Group activities 5 months 1 hr, 2 × week	Glycosuria HbA_1	NO -8%
Campaigne et al., 1984	9 children* (4 M/5 F)	10 children (2 M/8 F)	80% max HR 12 weeks 25 min, 3 × week	FBG HbA_1	-16% -10%
Rowland et al., 1985	13 children/adolescents (7 M/6 F)	—	60% HR reserve 12 weeks 1 hr, 3 × week	Glycosuria FBG	NO NO
Landt et al., 1985	9 adolescents (3 M/6 F)	5 adolescents (3 M/2 F)	160 HR 12 weeks 30 min, 3 × week	HbA_1	NO
Stratton et al., 1987	8 adolescents (4 M/4 F)	8 adolescents (4 M/4 F)	Aerobic activities 8 weeks 30-45 min, 3 × week	Glycosylated Serum Albumin FBG HbA_1	-16% NO NO

* < 11 years of age; HbA_1 = Glycosylated Hemoglobin; FBG = Fasting Blood Glucose; M = Males; F = Females; HR = Heart Rate

Table 3.2 Effects of Exercise on Glycemic Control in Adults with Type I Diabetes

Author	# Patients	Control subjects	Exercise program	Glycemic control	Effect
Costill et al., 1979	12 M	13 males Nondiabetic	60%-70% $\dot{V}O_2$max 10 weeks of running 30 min, 5 × week	FBG	-17%
Wallberg-Henriksson et al., 1982	9 M	—	60%-80% $\dot{V}O_2$max 16 weeks 1 hr, 2-3 × week	Glycosuria HbA$_1$	NO NO
Wallberg-Henriksson et al., 1984	10 M	10 males Nondiabetic	60%-80% $\dot{V}O_2$max 8 weeks 45 min, 3 × week	Mean BG HbA$_1$	NO NO
Zinman et al., 1984	13 adults (7 M/6F)	7 adults Nondiabetic (2 M/5 F)	60%-80% $\dot{V}O_2$max 12 weeks 45 min, 3 × week	FBG HbA$_1$	NO NO
Yki-Jarvinen et al., 1984	7 adults (6 M/1 F) Insulin pump therapy	6 adults with diabetes (4 M/2 F) 19 adults Nondiabetic	70% $\dot{V}O_2$max 6 weeks 30 min, 4 × week	Glycosuria Mean BG HbA$_1$	NO NO NO

BG = Blood glucose; HbA$_1$ = Glycosylated Hemoglobin; FBG = Fasting blood glucose; M = Males; F = Females

Most studies of adults with Type I diabetes have not shown improvements in HbA_1 with training (Wallberg-Henriksson, Gunnarsson, & Henriksson, 1982; Wallberg-Henriksson, Gunnarsson, Henriksson, Ostman, & Wahren, 1984; Yki-Jarvinen, DeFronzo, & Koivisto, 1984; Zinman, Zuniga-Guajardo, & Kelly, 1984). Wallberg-Henriksson and coworkers (Wallberg-Henriksson et al., 1982; Wallberg-Henriksson et al., 1984) found no change in blood glucose control as determined by HbA_1, home-monitored blood glucose levels, or glycosuria, in men after 8 to 16 weeks of physical training (see Figure 3.1). The subjects in these two studies had long disease duration and were considered in fair to good glycemic control. Zinman et al. (1984) studied aerobic capacity, blood glucose control, and dietary intake in adult men and women over 12 weeks of training, compared with a healthy control group. VO_2max increased significantly and similarly in the two groups. In the groups with diabetes, each exercise session resulted in a significant decrease in blood glucose levels, whereas HbA_1 did not change after the 12 weeks. There was no change in insulin dose or in the number of reported hypoglycemic occurrences during the study period. According to self report, caloric intake increased on exercise days. In a group of well-controlled patients on insulin pump treatment, Yki-Jarvinen et al. (1984) were unable to demonstrate any further improvement in blood glucose control with 12 weeks of training.

Bak, Jacobsen, Jorgensen, & Pedersen (1989) studied 4 male and 3 female young adult Type I patients (mean age 28 years) before and after 6 weeks of training three times per week. Maximal oxygen uptake increased and HbA_1 decreased slightly but significantly (7.9% ± 1.4% to 7.7% ± 1.5%) after training. Though statistically significant, the clinical significance of this decrease in HbA_1 is uncertain. Only one other reported exercise study in adults showed improved blood glucose control (Peterson, Jones, Esterly, Wantz, & Jackson, 1980). However, it was not possible to ascertain the effect of exercise alone in this study because training was started at the same time as subjects began a split-dose insulin regimen and self-monitored glucose determinations.

Very little information is available on resistance training in Type I diabetes. Strength training programs have been shown to improve insulin sensitivity and oral glucose tolerance (Hurley et al., 1984) as well as to improve lipid profiles in healthy adult men (Goldberg, Elliot, Schultz, & Koster, 1984). Durak, Jovanovic-Peterson, and Peterson (1990) demonstrated in 8 adult men with Type I diabetes that 10 min of resistance training three times a week resulted in significant strength gains accompanied by a significant decrease in glycosylated hemoglobin (6.9% ± 1.4% vs. 5.8% ± 0.9%; $p < 0.05$) and in total serum cholesterol. In the 152 exercise sessions there were 10 cases of hypoglycemia after exercise (blood glucose less than 3.64 mM), and all were corrected by 30g to 60g of oral glucose. It appears from this study that individuals with Type I diabetes can perform short sessions of resistance training without complications, and

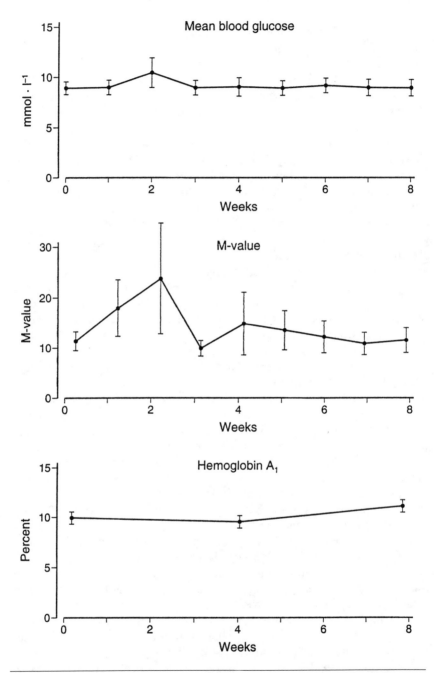

Figure 3.1 Blood glucose control assessed by home-monitored blood glucose (mean blood glucose and M-value) and HbA₁, before and during 8 weeks of training in men with IDDM.

the training may result in improvements in glucose control. Because this is the only work done on strength training in Type I diabetes, further study is warranted before recommendations can be made.

The supposed importance of regular exercise for long-term blood glucose control has not been well documented. The apparent discrepancy between some of the studies in children and adolescents and those in adults may not reflect a real difference in response to physical training. The study groups in general are not comparable; the children and adolescents who achieved improvements in HbA_1 had been in poorer blood glucose control before beginning exercise. In addition, they had diabetes of shorter duration, with perhaps some remaining residual insulin production, which in conjunction with increased insulin sensitivity may have affected the response (Campaigne & Gunnarsson, 1988). Though often studied, clinical indications of glucose metabolism may be less important than changes taking place at the cellular and subcellular level.

Insulin Sensitivity

It has been suggested that people with diabetes become more sensitive to exogenously administered insulin after physical training. Most studies cite no decrease or only a slight fall in insulin need during physical training, although Costill et al. (1979) noted a significant decrease in insulin dose during training. More recently, Bak, Jacobsen, Jorgensen, and Pedersen (1989) found a 12% decrease in how much insulin 7 Type I patients required ($43 \pm 9U/d$ to $38 \pm 8U/d$; $p < 0.05$) after 6 weeks of physical training.

Whole body insulin sensitivity, as assessed by the *glucose clamp* technique, is an acceptable measure of skeletal muscle insulin sensitivity when standard insulin infusion rates are used (DeFronzo, Tobin, & Andres, 1979). The effects of physical training on whole body insulin sensitivity are summarized in Table 3.3. Wallberg-Henriksson et al. (1982), Landt et al. (1985), and Yki-Jarvinen et al. (1984) have documented significant increases in insulin sensitivity as determined by the glucose clamp technique (Figure 3.2). All three studies reported approximately a 20% increase in insulin sensitivity after 6 to 16 weeks of physical training. Because well-trained, healthy controls have been found to have a higher insulin sensitivity when compared to their sedentary counterparts, this increase in insulin sensitivity brought about by physical training in individuals with diabetes appears to be a normal physiological adaptation. This increased insulin sensitivity is due in part to an increase in insulin action.

It has been suggested that the increased insulin sensitivity seen with acute exercise is attributable to the preceding acute exercise session.

Table 3.3 Effects of Exercise on Insulin Sensitivity in Type I Diabetes

Author	# Patients	Control subjects	Exercise program	Glycemic control	Effect
Wallberg-Henriksson et al., 1982	9 M	—	60%-80% $\dot{V}O_2$max 16 weeks 1 hr, 2-3 × week	Euglycemic clamp	+
Yki-Jarvinen et al., 1984	7 adults (6 M/1 F)	6 adults with diabetes (4 M/2 F) 19 adults Nondiabetic	70% $\dot{V}O_2$max 6 weeks 30 min, 4 × week	Euglycemic clamp	+
Landt et al., 1985	9 adolescents (3 M/6 F)	5 adolescents (3 M/2 F)	160 HR 12 weeks 30 min, 3 × week	Euglycemic clamp	+

+ = Increase; − = No effect; M = Males; F = Females; HR = Heart Rate

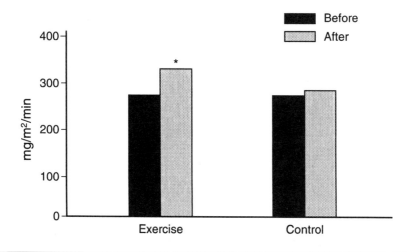

Figure 3.2   Insulin sensitivity determined by glucose utilization rate during the euglycemic clamp, before and after 8 weeks of exercise in Type I diabetes. Reprinted with permission from *Diabetes Care, 33,* 1985, p. 855. Copyright © 1985 by American Diabetes Association, Inc.

However, the effects of acute exercise last for about 24 hr, whereas the effects of physical training persist for several days. The following sections discuss muscular and cellular adaptations that could play a role in increased insulin sensitivity following physical training. Physical training appears to increase whole body tissue sensitivity to insulin. The precise mechanism behind increases in insulin sensitivity with physical training are currently unknown. The nature of the change in insulin sensitivity with physical training is probably related to glucose transport. Clarification of the mechanisms responsible for the increased insulin sensitivity with exercise in Type I diabetes is an important topic of current and future research.

Glucose Metabolism

Glucose uptake, transport, and metabolism are elevated after acute exercise and may persist after exercise as described in chapter 2 (page 38). It has been generally accepted that increases in glucose metabolism following exercise training are lost 48 hr after the last exercise session (Burstein et al., 1985; Heath et al., 1983). Acute and chronic exercise affect glucose metabolism in two different ways (Bonen, Tan, Megeney, & McDermott, 1992; Davis et al., 1986). Bonen et al. (1992) studied glucose metabolism in isolated soleus muscle from physically trained and untrained healthy rats following acute exercise. Acute exercise increased glycogenesis without altering glycolysis, whereas exercise training resulted in an increase in glycolysis that occurred only in the presence of insulin and lasted up to 96 hr after exercise. In combination with other data (Davis et al., 1986), these results suggest an effect of exercise training on the metabolism of skeletal muscle glucose beyond what was achieved in the last exercise session.

Glucose Transport

Glucose transport is considered the rate-limiting step to glucose utilization in skeletal muscle. Insulin-stimulated glucose transport into isolated skeletal muscle is decreased in experimentally induced diabetes (Wallberg-Henriksson & Holloszy, 1985). Both individuals with insulin-dependent diabetes and those with non-insulin-dependent diabetes exhibit peripheral insulin resistance (DeFronzo, Hendler, & Simonson, 1982; Olefsky, Kolterman, & Scarlett, 1982), resulting in a deterioration in glucose homeostasis. The underlying mechanisms responsible for peripheral insulin resistance are not well known. The state of insulinization, nutritional status, and muscle activity demonstrably are the most important factors related to glucose transport into skeletal muscle (Wallberg-Henriksson & Wahren, 1989).

Glucose tolerance is increased for several days after a single bout of exercise. This increase is partially attributable to greater glucose uptake by skeletal muscle to replenish depleted glycogen stores (Fell, Terblanche, Ivy, Young, & Holloszy, 1982). Frequent exercise sessions prevent the decreased contraction-induced glucose transport usually seen in insulin-deficient diabetic rats (Wallberg-Henriksson, 1986). These findings clearly demonstrate that muscular activity is directly involved in regulating the glucose transport system.

The entry of glucose into skeletal muscle takes place by means of a system of protein transport molecules termed glucose carriers or transporters. The Glut 1 isoform is thought to be primarily involved in glucose transport under basal conditions, whereas Glut 4 is insulin stimulated and affected by exercise and muscle contraction (Barnard & Youngren, 1992). Exercise may affect glucose transport independent of insulin (see chapter 2, pages 39-40).

Acute exercise increases glucose transport by recruiting Glut 4 transporters to the plasma membrane from an intracellular pool. The initial response may involve calcium, but the mechanism for the increased insulin sensitivity's lasting up to a day after acute exercise is unknown. Recently, an increase in the content of Glut 4 transporters in the sarcolemma of skeletal muscle after exercise training has been reported (Barnard and Youngren, 1992).

Ploug et al. (1990) reported an increase in insulin-stimulated glucose uptake in rats after 10 weeks of swim training. Goodyear, Hirshman, Valyou, and Horton (1992) found a similar increase in glucose transport that resulted from an increase in the activity and quantity of Glut 4 translocated to the sacrolemma. These researchers also noted an increase in Glut 4 mRNA with exercise training (Wake et al., 1991). Rodnick,

Holloszy, Mondon, and James (1990) found an increase in Glut 4 concentration in plantaris muscle with no change in soleus muscle after 6 weeks of voluntary treadmill running and attributed the increase to the soleus being primarily slow-twitch oxidative muscle and the plantaris a mixed-fiber muscle. Very little research has been done on glucose transporters in humans; however, Houmard et al. (1991) revealed no change in Glut 4 after acute exercise and a marked increase following physical training. Thus, Glut 4 has been shown to increase with physical training. The increase appears to occur in specific muscle groups and may be related to fiber type. Further evidence points to an increase in Glut 4 mRNA and protein.

Physical training, then, produces the following increases in glucose transport:

- Glucose transport in specific muscle groups and fiber types increases.
- The quantity of Glut 4 transporters translocated to the sacrolemma increases.
- Glut 4 activity increases.
- Glut 4 mRNA increases.
- Glut 4 protein increases.

From these studies we can conclude that alterations in glucose are present in individuals with diabetes. Glucose transport improves after repeated sessions of muscle contraction in these individuals, just as glucose transport is increased after physical training in healthy animals and humans. Further work needs to be done on the effects of physical training on glucose transport in diabetes.

Insulin Binding

As mentioned previously, insulin binding may be an important step in the regulation of glucose transport. Increased insulin binding to *erythrocytes* and *monocytes* has been found in highly trained, healthy individuals (Burstein et al., 1985; Heath et al., 1983). Increased insulin binding to monocytes and erythrocytes has also been found after acute exercise in Type I patients (Pederson, Beck-Nielsen, & Heding, 1980).

The long-term effects of exercise on insulin binding were not well documented until recently, probably because of a lack of consistency in tissues studied and methodologies utilized. Reports of insulin binding to erythrocytes after physical training are conflicting (Baevre, Sovik, Wisnes, & Heirvang, 1985; Yki-Jarvinen et al., 1984). It is now known that erythrocytes and monocytes do not provide a good index of insulin binding in skeletal muscle, the tissue most likely affected by exercise. Bak, Jacobsen, Jorgensen, and Pedersen (1989) demonstrated an altered number of insulin receptors in Type I patients compared with healthy controls at baseline. These authors cited no change in insulin receptor number or insulin binding in insulin receptors derived from skeletal muscle after 6 weeks of physical training (see the section on muscle enzyme activity on this page). Tan and Bonen (1987) have shown that insulin binding to soleus muscle is increased after physical training in healthy mice.

Skeletal Muscle Metabolism

Contraction of skeletal muscle is one of the principle components of exercise, and skeletal muscle is the primary tissue that shows adaptations to physical training. These adaptations are manifest in several measurable responses.

Muscle Enzyme Activities

Costill et al. (1979) have reported increases in muscle lipoprotein lipase (LpL), succinate dehydrogenase, and hexokinase activity after 12 weeks of training in men with Type I diabetes. However, Lithell, Krokiweski, and Kiens (1985) have reported no change in muscle LpL activity after training, a finding perhaps related to the absence of an increase in skeletal muscle capillarization. Thus, changes in skeletal muscle capillarization may be necessary for discernable improvements in muscle LpL.

Wallberg-Henriksson et al. (1982) noted changes in mitochondrial oxidative enzyme activity similar to those of Costill et al. (1979) after 16 weeks of training in adult men with diabetes. In a subsequent study, Wallberg-Henriksson et al. (1984) evaluated the effects of training on skeletal muscle enzyme activity and muscle capillarization. In the latter study, hexokinase activity was lower in the group with diabetes before training, compared with healthy controls. Exercise training resulted in an increase in hexokinase activity in the patient group (+28%), bringing it up to a level comparable to the control group, in which it increased only 5% with training. Lactate dehydrogenase activity before training was significantly higher in the group with diabetes and tended to decrease with training, whereas it remained unchanged in the control group. Skeletal muscle oxidative capacity increased similarly in the two groups as evidenced by significant increases in citrate synthase and succinate dehydrogenase activities. Saltin, Houston, Nygaard, Graham, and Wahren (1979) have also reported reduced levels of hexokinase and elevated levels of lactate dehydrogenase activity in skeletal muscle of Type I patients, compared with normal control subjects. Insulin-stimulated tyrosine kinase activity in skeletal muscle has been shown to decrease or remain unchanged after physical training in rats (Dohm, Sinha, & Caro, 1987; Santos, Mondon, Reaven, & Azhar, 1989). Findings on muscle enzyme activity with physical training in Type I diabetes are summarized in Table 3.4.

Table 3.4   The Effects of Physical Training on Skeletal Muscle Enzyme Activity in Type I Diabetes

LpL*	Increased or unchanged (possibly related to capillarization)
Succinate dehydrogenase	Increased
Hexokinase	Low before training Increased with training
Lactate dehydrogenase	Elevated before training Decreased with training
Citrate synthase	Increased
Glycogen synthase	Increased

*Lipoprotein lipase

Glycogen Synthesis

At least part of the increase in insulin sensitivity found to occur with physical training appears attributable to the resynthesis of depleted muscle glycogen stores (Bogardus et al., 1983; Devlin & Horton, 1985). Glycogen storage capacity is reduced in the skeletal muscle of patients with insulin-dependent diabetes mellitus (Bak et al., 1989; Saltin et al., 1979; Wallberg-Henriksson et al., 1982). Glycogen storage capacity has been shown to improve with regular exercise, due to increases in skeletal muscle enzyme activity (Bak et al., 1989; Wallberg-Henriksson et al., 1982). Thus, Bak et al. have examined insulin receptor function and glycogen synthase activity in the skeletal muscle of diabetic patients before and after 6 weeks of physical training. At baseline, glycogen synthase activity and insulin receptor number were significantly lower in diabetic subjects, when compared with a control group without diabetes. There was no difference between the two groups in the half-maximal activation constant of glucose-6-phosphate. Both basal and insulin-stimulated receptor kinase activities were identical in the two groups. After physical training in those with diabetes, $\dot{V}O_2$max increased significantly (45.7 ± 7.4 ml/kg/min to 48.9 ± 9.0 ml/kg/min; $p < 0.05$), and, as previously mentioned, HbA_1 and insulin requirements decreased. Maximal glycogen synthase activity increased by 15%, with no change occurring in glucose-6-phosphate (see Figure 3.3). After physical training, both the number of insulin receptors recovered and the receptor kinase activity were unaltered from baseline. Thus, in Type I subjects insulin receptor kinase was normal at baseline whereas insulin receptor binding in skeletal muscle was impaired, as was the capacity for glycogen storage. Glycogen storage capacity, as evidenced by glycogen synthase activity, improved, but insulin receptor function was unchanged after 6 weeks of physical training.

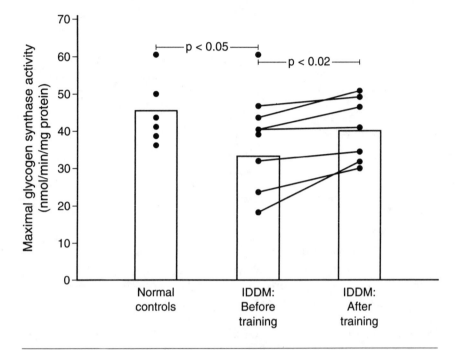

Figure 3.3   Individual and mean maximal glycogen synthase activity in muscle biopsies of 7 nondiabetic subjects and 7 IDDM patients before and after training. The glycogen synthase activity was determine in the presence of 0.13 m mol/L UDP-(U-14C) glucose and 6.7 m mol/L G6P.

From "Insulin Receptor Function and Glycogen Synthase Activity in Skeletal Muscle Biopsies From Patients With Insulin-Dependent Diabetes Mellitus" by J.F. Bak, U.K. Jacobsen, F.S. Jorgensen, and O. Pedersen, 1989, *Journal of Clinical Endocrinology and Metabolism*, **69**, p. 161. Copyright 1989 byThe Endocrine Society. Reprinted by permission.

Muscle Capillarization

Increases in skeletal muscle capillarization with physical training are well documented in healthy subjects (Andersen & Henriksson, 1977). Specifically, increases in mean capillary density (capillaries per fiber area) have been found to occur in conjunction with increases in $\dot{V}O_2$max. Wallberg-Henriksson et al. (1984) found that individuals with diabetes did not increase mean capillary density of the muscle, whereas a healthy control group increased capillary density significantly after 16 weeks of training. Interestingly, when stratifying the patient group by duration of disease it was found that people with diabetes of shorter duration (mean 11 years) showed increases in capillarization with training, whereas those with diabetes of longer duration (mean 18 years) did not. This may be evidence that the "normal" adaptation of skeletal muscle capillarization to physical training becomes more difficult to achieve the longer the duration of diabetes. Saltin et al. (1979) noted a lower capillary density in insulin-dependent patients compared with control subjects of similar aerobic capacity, and Lithell, Krokiweski, and Kiens (1985) also reported a lack of response in muscle capillarization to training. Thus, muscle capillarization and increases in capillarization with physical training may be related to the duration of diabetes.

Serum Lipids and Lipoproteins

Individuals with insulin-dependent diabetes exhibit accelerated athero-sclerosis, generally after 10 to 15 years duration of diabetes (Ganda, 1980). Abnormal blood lipids may contribute to this high incidence of atherosclerotic development among individuals with diabetes. Physical training has been shown to improve lipid profiles in healthy subjects (Haskell, 1984; Hietanen, 1982; Wood et al., 1976). The improvements include increases in high-density lipoprotein cholesterol (HDL-C) and decreased concentrations of triglycerides, low-density lipoprotein cholesterol (LDL-C), or both. Thus, the effects of regular exercise on lipid profiles in those with diabetes may have important clinical implications. The effects of physical training on blood lipids in patients with Type 1 diabetes are summarized in Table 3.5. After training, serum triglycerides (Costill et al., 1979; Larsson, Persson, Sterky, & Thoren, 1964b) and total cholesterol (Costill et al., Wallberg-Henriksson et al., 1982) have been reported to decrease, and HDL-C/total cholesterol ratio (Costill et al., Yki-Jarvinen et al., 1984) to increase. Others, however, have reported no change in either cholesterol or triglycerides after training (Baevre, Sovik, Wisnes, & Heirvang, 1985; Campaigne et al., 1985). LDL-C has been found to decrease significantly in adolescent males and females with Type I diabetes after 12 weeks of physical training (Campaigne et al.).

It appears that the most profound effects of physical training on lipid profiles in Type I subjects is on total cholesterol, triglycerides, and LDL-C. The absence of an absolute change in HDL-C in these patients contrasts with most reports on the effects of physical training on lipid profiles in healthy subjects (Haskell, 1984; Hietanen, 1982; Wood et al., 1976). Type I patients often have high HDL-C levels initially, which may affect their ability to increase HDL-C in response to exercise—in healthy subjects the lower the HDL-C levels at baseline the greater the increase with physical training (Williams et al., 1983).

In a cross-sectional study Gunnarsson, Wallberg-Henriksson, Rossner, and Wahren (1987) examined the relationship between serum lipoprotein levels, glycemic control, and physical fitness in female Type I patients. Subjects were divided into three groups based on glycemic control: good (HbA$_1$ 9.5%), acceptable (HbA$_1$ 9.6% to 10.9%), and poor (HbA$_1$ 11.0%).

Table 3.5 Effects of Exercise on Blood Lipids in Type I Diabetes

Author	# Patients	Control subjects	Exercise program	Serum lipids	Effect
Larsson et al., 1964	6 adolescents (6 M)	6 adolescents (6 M) Healthy controls	Gymnastics 5 months 1 hr, 1 × week	TG TC	Lower TG
Costill et al., 1979	12 adults (12 M)	13 adults (13 M) Healthy controls	60%-70% $\dot{V}O_2$max 10 weeks running 30 min, 5 × week	TG TC	Lower TG Lower TC
Wallberg-Henriksson et al., 1982	9 adults (9 M)	—	60%-80% $\dot{V}O_2$max 16 weeks 1 hr, 2-3 × week	TG, TC LDL-C HDL-C	Lower TC Higher HDL/TC
Campaigne et al., 1985	9 adolescents (3 M/6 F)	5 adolescents (3 M/2 F)	160 HR 12 weeks 45 min, 3 × week	TG, TC LDL-C HDL-C	Lower LDL

LDL-C = Low-Density Lipoprotein Cholesterol; HDL-C = High-Density Lipoprotein Cholesterol; TG = Triglycerides; TC = Total Cholesterol; M = Males; F = Females

Those in good control were found to have the lowest triglyceride concentrations, mainly attributed to lower VLDL-triglyceride. The patients in good control also had higher HDL-C and HDL 2 cholesterol concentrations, whereas HDL 3 cholesterol was similar in all groups. When patients were grouped by $\dot{V}O_2$max, the group with higher aerobic capacity also had lower triglycerides, consistent with a lower LDL fraction. HDL 2 cholesterol and the HDL 2/HDL 3 ratio were found to be significantly elevated in subjects with high $\dot{V}O_2$max. Adding HbA_1 to the multiple regression analysis with $\dot{V}O_2$max and the lipid and lipoprotein parameters did not further explain the variability of the lipid fraction under study. These authors concluded that both good glycemic control and high aerobic capacity may be important for favorable lipid status in patients with Type I diabetes.

Epidemiological Evidence

Only limited information is currently available regarding the long-term effects of exercise in patients with Type I diabetes. Data from the Joslin Clinic on 48 patients at 25-year follow-up indicate that men who developed complications from the disease reported a lower frequency of physical activity compared to those who were free of complications (Chazan, Balodimos, Ryan, & Marble, 1970). LaPorte, Dorman, & Tajima (1986) observed a lower incidence of macrovascular disease in patients with insulin-dependent diabetes who engaged in team sports in high school and college compared with their sedentary counterparts. These investigators also reported a lower incidence of mortality in the physically active group after 25 years. More recently, Moy et al. (1993) reported on a cohort of 548 diabetes patients followed over 7 years. Baseline physical activity was inversely related to risk of mortality during the 7-year period. Males expending less than 1,000 kcal per week had a threefold greater risk of death than those expending more than 2,000 kcal per week. These findings were similar, but not as evident, in females. These results are similar to the findings of Paffenbarger, Wing, and Hyde (1978) in healthy controls. These findings further support that even a moderate level of activity performed on a regular basis is beneficial in improving longevity in individuals with diabetes.

Summary

Regular exercise may have little or no effect on long-term blood glucose control, but exercise does improve insulin sensitivity and may be beneficial in improving blood lipids and glycogen-storage capacity in patients with Type I diabetes. Though clinical correlates of glucose control may not be improved by regular exercise, research on subcellular increases in glucose transport and glucose metabolism appear beneficial. In addition, there is some epidemiological evidence to suggest that individuals with Type I diabetes who exercise throughout life may develop fewer complications and live longer lives than those who have not exercised.

References

Andersen, P., & Henriksson, J. (1977). Capillary supply of the quadriceps femoris muscle of man: Adaptive response to exercise. *Journal of Physiology, 270*, 677-690.

Baevre, H., Sovik, O., Wisnes, A., & Heirvang, E. (1985). Metabolic responses to physical training in young insulin-dependent diabetics. *Scandinavian Journal of Clinical and Laboratory Investigation, 45*, 109-114.

Bak, J.F., Jacobsen, U.K., Jorgensen, F.S., & Pedersen, O. (1989). Insulin receptor function and glycogen synthase activity in skeletal muscle biopsies from patients with insulin dependent diabetes mellitus: Effects of physical training. *Journal of Clinical Endocrinology and Metabolism, 69*, 158-164.

Barnard, R.J., & Youngren, J.F. (1992). Regulation of glucose transport in skeletal muscle. *FASEB Journal, 6*(14), 3238-3244.

Bogardus, C., Thuillez, P., Ravussin, E., Vasquez, B., Narimiga, M.F., & Azhar, S. (1983). Effect of muscle glycogen depletion on in vivo insulin action in men. *Journal of Clinical Investigation, 72*, 1605-1610.

Bonen, A., Tan, M.H., Megeney, L.A., & McDermott, J.C. (1992). Persistence of glucose metabolism after exercise in trained and untrained soleus muscle. *Diabetes Care, 15*, 1694-1700.

Burstein, R., Polychronakos, C., Toews, C.J., MacDougall, J.D., Guyda, H.J., & Posner, B.I. (1985). Acute reversal of the enhanced insulin action in trained athletes. Association with insulin receptor changes. *Diabetes, 34*, 756-760.

Campaigne, B.N., Gilliam, T.B., Spencer, M.L., Lampman, R.M., & Schork, M.A. (1984). Effects of a physical activity program on metabolic control and cardiovascular fitness in children with insulin dependent diabetes mellitus. *Diabetes Care, 7*, 57-62.

Campaigne, B.N., & Gunnarsson, R. (1988). The effects of physical training in people with insulin-dependent diabetes. *Diabetic Medicine, 5*, 429-433.

Campaigne, B.N., Landt, K.W., Mellies, M.J., James, F.W., Glueck, C.J., & Sperling, M.A. (1985). The effects of physical training on blood lipid profiles in adolescents with insulin dependent diabetes mellitus. *Physician Sports Medicine,* **13,** 83-89.

Charron, M.J., Brosius, F.C., III, Alper, S.L., Lodish, H.F. (1989). A novel glucose transport protein expressed predominantly in insulin-responsive tissues. *Proceeding of the National Academy of Sciences USA,* **86,** 2235-2239.

Chazan, B.I., Balodimos, M.C., Ryan, J.R., & Marble, A. (1970). Twenty-five to forty-five years of diabetes with and without vascular complications. *Diabetologia,* **6,** 565-569.

Compagnucci, P., Cartechini, N.G., Bolli, G., DeFeo, P., Santeusanio, F., & Brunettio, P. (1981). The importance of determining irreversibly glycosylated hemoglobin in diabetes. *Diabetes,* **30,** 607-612.

Costill, D.L., Cleary, P., Find, W., Foster, C., Ivy, J.L., & Witzmann, F. (1979). Training adaptations in skeletal muscles of juvenile diabetics. *Diabetes,* **28I,** 818-822.

Dahl-Jorgensen, K., Meen, H.D., Hanssen, K.R.F., & Genaes, O.A.A. (1980). The effect of exercise on diabetic control and hemoglobin A (HbA₁) in children. *Acta Paediatrica Scandinavica,* **283** (Suppl. 283), 53-56.

Davis, T.A., Klahr, S., Tegtmeyer, E.D., Osborne, D.F., Howard, T.L., & Karl, I.E. (1986). Glucose metabolism in epitrochlearis muscle of acutely exercised and trained rats. *American Journal of Physiology,* **250,** E137-E143.

DeFronzo, A., Tobin, J.D., & Andres, R. (1979). Glucose clamp technique: A method for quantifying insulin secretion and resistance. *American Journal of Physiology,* **237** E214-E223.

DeFronzo, R.A., Hendler, R., & Simonson, D. (1982). Insulin resistance is a prominent feature of insulin-dependent diabetes. *Diabetes,* **31,** 795-801.

Devlin, J.T., & Horton, E.S. (1985). Effects of prior high intensity exercise on glucose metabolism in normal and insulin resistant men. *Diabetes,* **34,** 973-978.

Dohm, G.L., Sinha, M.K., & Caro, J.F. (1987). Insulin receptor binding and protein kinase activity in muscles of trained rats. *American Journal of Physiology,* **252,** E170-E175.

Douen, A.G., Rastogi, S., Cartee, G.D., Holloszy, J.O., Ramlal, T., Bilan, P.J., Vranic, M., & Klip, A. (1990). Exercise induces recruitment of the "insulin-responsive glucose transporter." *Journal of Biological Chemistry,* **265,** 13427-13430.

Durak, E.P., Jovanovik-Peterson, J., & Peterson, C.M. (1990). Randomized crossover study of effect of resistance training on glycemic control, muscular strength, and cholesterol in Type I diabetic men. *Diabetes Care,* **13,** 1039-1043.

Fell, R.D., Terblanche, S.E., Ivy, J.L., Young, J.C., & Holloszy, J.O. (1982). Effect of muscle glycogen content on glucose uptake following exercise. *Journal of Applied Physiology, 51*, 434-437.

Ganda, O.P. (1980). Pathogenesis of macrovascular disease in the human diabetic. *Diabetes, 29*, 931-942.

Goldberg, L., Elliot, D.L., Schultz, R.W., & Kloster, F.E. (1984). Changes in lipid and lipoprotein levels after weight training. *Journal of the American Medical Association, 252*, 504-506.

Goodyear, L.J., Hirshman, M.F., Smith, R.J., & Horton, E.S. (1991). Glucose transporter number, activity, and isoform content in plasma membranes of red and white skeletal muscle. *American Journal of Physiology, 261*, E556-E561.

Goodyear, L.J., Hirshman, M.F., Valyou, P.M., & Horton, E.S. (1992). Glucose transporter number, function and subcellular distribution in rat skeletal muscle after exercise training. *Diabetes, 41*, 1091-1099.

Gunnarsson, R., Wallberg-Henriksson, H., Rossner, S., & Wahren, J. (1987). Serum lipid and lipoprotein levels in female Type I diabetics: Relationships to aerobic capacity and glycaemic control. *Diabetes and Metabolism, 13*, 417-421.

Haskell, W.L. (1984). Exercise induced changes in lipids and lipoprotein levels. *Preventive Medicine, 13*, 23-34.

Heath, G.W., Gavin, J.R., III, Hinderliter, J.M., Hagberg, J.M., Bloomfield, S.A., & Holloszy, J.O. (1983). Effects of exercise and lack of exercise on glucose tolerance and insulin sensitivity. *Journal of Applied Physiology, 55*, 512-517.

Hietanen, E. (Ed.) (1982). *Regulation of serum lipids by physical exercise.* Boca Raton, Florida: CRC Press.

Houmard, J.A., Egan, P.C., Neufer, P.D., Friedman, J.E., Wheeler, W.S., Israel, R.G., & Dohm, G.L. (1991). Elevated skeletal muscle glucose transporter levels in exercise-trained middle-aged men. *American Journal of Physiology, 261*, E437-E443.

Hurley, F.B., Seals, D.R., Ehsani, A.A., Cartier, L.J., Dalsky, G.P., Hagberg, J.M., & Holloszy, J.O. (1984). Effects of high intensity strength training on cardiovascular function. *Medicine and Science in Sports and Exercise, 16*, 483-488.

Klip, A., Marette, A., Dimitrakoudis, D., Ramlal, T., Giacca, A., Shi, Z.Q., & Vranic, M. (1992). Effect of diabetes on glucoregulation. From glucose transporters to glucose metabolism in vivo. *Diabetes Care, 15*, 1747-1766.

Landt, K.W., Campaigne, B.N., James, F.W., & Sperling, M.A. (1985). Effects of exercise training on insulin sensitivity in adolescents with Type I diabetes. *Diabetes Care, 8*, 461-465.

Langfort, J., Budohoski, L., & Newsholme, E.A. (1988). Effect of various types of acute exercise and exercise training on the insulin sensitivity of rat soleus muscle measured in vitro. *Pflugers Arch,* **412**, 101-105.

LaPorte, R.E., Dorman, J.S., & Tajima, N. (1986). Pittsburgh insulin-dependent diabetes mellitus morbidity and mortality study; physical activity and diabetic complications. *Pediatrics,* **78**, 1027-1033.

Larsson, Y., Persson, B., Sterky, G., & Thoren, C. (1964a). Functional adaptation to rigorous training and exercise in diabetic and non-diabetic adolescents. *Journal of Applied Physiology,* **19**, 629-635.

Larsson, Y., Persson, B., Sterky, G., & Thoren, C. (1964b). Effects of exercise on blood lipids in juvenile diabetics. *Lancet,* **i**, 350-355.

Larsson, Y.A.A., Sterky, G.C.C., Ekengren, K.E.K., & Moller, T.G.H.P. (1962). Physical fitness and the influence of training in diabetic adolescent girls. *Diabetes,* **11**, 109-117.

Lithell, H., Krokiweski, M., & Kiens, B. (1985). Non-response of muscle capillary density and lipoprotein-lipase activity to regular training in diabetic patients. *Diabetes Research,* **2**, 17-21.

Moy, C.S., Songer, T.J., LaPorte, R.E., Dorman, J.S., Kriska, A.M., Orchard, T.J., Becker, D.J., & Drash, A.L. (1993). Insulin-dependent diabetes mellitus, physical activity, and death. *American Journal of Epidemiology,* **137**, 74-81.

Olefsky, J.M., Kolterman, O.G., & Scarlett, J.A. (1982). Insulin action and resistance in obesity and noninsulin-dependent Type II diabetes mellitus. *American Journal of Physiology,* **243**, E15-E30.

Paffenbarger, R.S., Jr., Wing, A.L., & Hyde, R.T. (1978). Physical activity as an index of heart attack risk in college alumni. *American Journal of Epidemiology,* **108**, 161-175.

Pedersen, O., Beck-Nielsen, H., & Heding, L. (1980). Increased insulin receptors after exercise in patients with insulin dependent diabetes mellitus. *New England Journal of Medicine,* **302**, 886-892.

Peterson, C.M., Jones, R.L., Esterly, J.A., Wantz, G.E., Jackson, R.L. (1980). Changes in basement membrane thickening and pulse volume concomitant with improved glucose control and exercise in patients with insulin dependent diabetes mellitus. *Diabetes Care,* **3**, 586-589.

Ploug, T., Stallknecht, B.M., Pederson, O., Kahn, B.B., Ohkuwa, T., Vinten, J., & Galbo, H. (1990). Effect of endurance training on glucose transport capacity and glucose transporter expression in rat skeletal muscle. *American Journal of Physiology,* **259**, E778-E786.

Rodnick, K.J., Henriksen, E.J., James, D.E., & Holloszy, J.O. (1992). Exercise training, glucose transporters, and glucose transport in rat skeletal muscles. *American Journal of Physiology,* **262**, C9-C14.

Rodnick, K.J., Holloszy, J.O., Mondon, C.E., & James, D.E. (1990). Effects of exercise training on insulin-regulatable glucose-transporter protein levels in rat skeletal muscle. *Diabetes,* **39**, 1425-1429.

Rowland, T.W., Swadba, L.A., Biggs, D.E., Burke, E.J., & Ritter, E.O. (1985). Glycemic control with physical training in insulin dependent diabetes mellitus. *American Journal of Diseases of Children*, **139**, 307-309.

Saltin, B., Houston, M., Nygaard, E., Graham, T., & Wahren, J. (1979). Muscle fiber characteristics in healthy men and patients with juvenile diabetes. *Diabetes*, **28**(Suppl. I), 9399.

Sane, T., Helve, E., Pelkonen, R., & Koivisto, V.A. (1988). The adjustment of diet and insulin dose during long-term endurance exercise in Type I (insulin-dependent) diabetic men. *Diabetologia*, **31**, 35-40.

Santos, R.F., Mondon, C.E., Reaven, G.M., & Azhar, S. (1989). Effects of exercise training on the relationship between insulin binding and insulin-stimulated tyrosine kinase activity in rat skeletal muscle. *Metabolism*, **38**, 376-386.

Stratton, E.L., Wilson, D.P., Endres, R.K., & Goldstein, D.E. (1987). Improved glycemic control after supervised 8 week exercise program in insulin dependent diabetic adolescents. *Diabetes Care*, **10**, 589-593.

Sushruta, S.C.S. (1938). *Vaidya Jayayaji Trikamji Acharia*. Bombay, India: Nirnyar Sagar.

Tan, M.H., & Bonen, A. (1987). Effect of exercise training on insulin binding and glucose metabolism in mouse soleus muscle. *Canadian Journal of Physiology and Pharmacology*, **65**, 2231-2234.

Wake, S.A., Sowden, J.A., Storlien, L.H., James, D.E., Clark, P.E., Shine, J., Chisholm, D.J., & Kraegen, W.E. (1991). Effects of exercise training and dietary manipulation on insulin-regulatable glucose-transporter mRNA in rat muscle. *Diabetes*, **40**, 275-279.

Wallberg-Henriksson, H. (1986). Repeated exercise regulates glucose transport capacity in skeletal muscle. *Acta Physiologica Scandinavica*, **127**, 39-43.

Wallberg-Henriksson, H., Gunnarsson, R., & Henriksson, J. (1982). Increased peripheral insulin sensitivity and muscle mitochondrial enzymes but unchanged glycemic control in Type I diabetics after physical training. *Diabetes*, **31**, 1022-1650.

Wallberg-Henriksson, H., Gunnarsson, R., Henriksson, J., Ostman, J., & Wahren, J. (1984). Influence of physical training on formation of muscle capillaries in Type I diabetes. *Diabetes*, **33**, 851-857.

Wallberg-Henriksson, H., & Holloszy, J.O. (1985). Activation of glucose transport in diabetic muscle: Responses to contraction and insulin. *American Journal of Physiology*, **249**, C233-C237.

Wallberg-Henriksson, H., & Wahren, J. (1989). Effects of nutrition and diabetes mellitus on the regulation of metabolic fuels during exercise. *American Journal of Clinical Nutrition*, **411**(Suppl. 5), 938-943.

Williams, P.T., Wood, P.D., Krauss, R.M., Haskell, W.L., Vranizan, K.M., Blair, S.N., Terry, R., & Farquhar, J.W. (1983). Does weight loss cause the exercise induced increase in plasma high density lipoproteins? *Atherosclerosis*, **913**(47), 173-185.

Wood, P.D., Haskell, W.L., Klein, H., Lewis, S., Stern, M.P., & Farquhar, J.W. (1976). The distribution of plasma lipoproteins in middle-aged male runners. *Metabolism*, **11**, 1249-1257.

Yki-Jarvinen, H., DeFronzo, P., & Koivisto, V.A. (1984). Normalization of insulin sensitivity in Type I diabetic subjects by physical training during insulin pump therapy. *Diabetes Care*, **7**, 520-527.

Zinman, B., Zuniga-Guajardo, S., & Kelly, D. (1984). Comparison of the acute and long-term effects of exercise on glucose control in Type I diabetes. *Diabetes Care*, **7**, 515-519.

Chapter 4

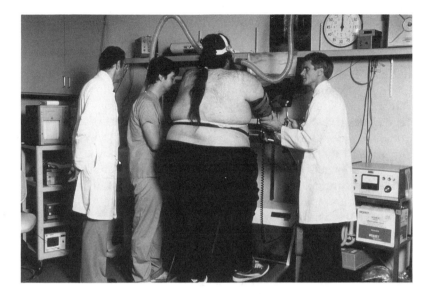

Metabolic and Physiologic Responses to Acute Exercise in Type II Diabetes

The various aspects of acute exercise, such as its duration and intensity, contribute to the unique responses of the individual metabolically, cardiovascularly, neurally, and hormonally. The balance of insulin, glucagon, and catecholamines affects the availability of metabolic fuel for muscular contractions. For individuals with Type II diabetes, glycemic, neural, cardiovascular, and other factors may alter what would be considered a normal response to acute exercise. This chapter will focus on the various aspects of the metabolic profile and physiologic environment of individuals with Type II diabetes and how these factors may influence his or her response to exercise.

Substrate Utilization in People Without Diabetes

Acute exercise in people without diabetes results in rapid metabolic, cardiovascular, neural, and hormonal responses to ensure adequate mobilization, usage, and redistribution of energy sources (Coggan, 1991). At-rest glucose utilization represents about 10% of skeletal muscle's energy requirement, and 85% to 90% of energy comes from free fatty acids (FFA) (Gollnick, 1985). Resting muscle utilization of amino acids is limited, representing only 1% to 2% of energy sources. These percentages change with exercise depending on its duration and intensity. As exercise begins, blood is shunted from inactive sites to contracting muscle and, at the same time, to the skin to help with the cooling process. This change in blood flow alters energy sources at the active muscle sites. As a result, substrate utilization differs markedly during exercise, compared with rest, and it remains altered throughout and following the exercise session. Energy provided to skeletal muscle at the onset of exercise comes from high-energy phosphate compounds such as adenosine triphosphate and phosphocreatine. The regulation of glucose utilization in human skeletal muscle during this initial phase is limited by phosphorylation (Katz, Sahlin, & Broberg, 1991). Muscle glycogen and lipid stores within the muscle serve as an early source of energy until adequate blood-borne substrates are available (Hermansen, Hultman, & Saltin, 1967). As exercise continues past 3 min, circulating glucose from hepatic sources and FFA mobilized from adipose sites become more important energy sources (Ahlborg, Felig, Hagenfeldt, Hendler, & Wahren, 1974). Blood glucose uptake by contracting muscle may account for 8% to 14% of the energy source during the first 10 min of moderate exercise (Wahren, Felig, Ahlborg, & Jorfeldt, 1971). During periods of exercise lasting 40 to 50 min, glucose energy sources may represent 20% to 30% of total muscle oxidative metabolism (Henriksson, 1977; Wahren et al., 1971). Periods of exercise lasting 90 to 180 min result in a greater glucose utilization, representing 35% to 40% of total oxidative metabolism of working muscle.

The intensity of exercise effort also greatly influences substrate utilization by contracting muscle. During moderate exercise, energy utilization is balanced between glucose and FFA sources. At low intensity of effort, plasma glucose levels remain stable or decrease. At high exercise intensity, energy from glucose oxidation is the principal source of substrate utilization. Blood glucose levels initially increase and may eventually decline during prolonged exercise as hepatic stores are depleted. In terms of local stores, muscle glycogen can be markedly reduced during high-intensity exercise resulting in 65% to 85% of $\dot{V}O_2$max that lasts up to 2 to 3 hr. During this time, blood-borne substrates account for 90% of the energy source. In comparison with moderate-intensity exercise, FFA contribute more to oxidative metabolism of exercising muscle during prolonged periods at low intensities (Ahlborg et al., 1974).

Under normal metabolic conditions, hepatic glucose production increases to replenish blood glucose, and thus euglycemia is maintained. This is initially accomplished primarily by *glycogenolysis*, and as exercise continues gluconeogenesis becomes more prominent (Ahlborg et al., 1974). The main substrates for gluconeogenesis during prolonged exercise are lactate, alanine, and glycerol (Wahren et al., 1971). The interaction of glucagon and insulin controls hepatic glycogenolysis and gluconeogenesis (Wasserman, Spalding, Bracy, Lacy, & Cherrington, 1989; Wasserman, Spalding, Lacy, Colburn, Goldstein, & Cherrington, 1989), whereas both the fall in insulin and increased epinephrine levels control FFA fluxes and muscle glycogenolysis. As exercise continues, muscle and hepatic glycogen stores become depleted (Price, Rothman, Avison, Buonamico, & Shulman, 1991), and blood glucose concentrations decrease (Vranic & Berger, 1979). Plasma glucose utilization decreases, insulin levels continue to decline, counterregulatory hormone levels continue to increase, and FFA resulting from lipolysis become increasingly more important as energy sources (Ahlborg et al., 1974; Franz, 1987). Nonworking muscles assist by taking up and oxidizing significant amounts of lactate (Lindinger, Heigenhauser, McKelvie, & Jones, 1990).

Increased muscle uptake of FFA during the first 10 min of exercise results in a transient fall in blood FFA concentrations if large-muscle groups are involved (Hagenfeldt, Wahren, Pernow, & Raf, 1972). As exercise continues, lipolysis progressively increases blood FFA levels to reach a steady state at approximately 30 to 40 min of moderate exercise intensity (Hagenfeldt & Wahren, 1968). At 40 to 90 min of exercise, FFA contribute 37% to 38% to oxidative metabolism. From 180 to 240 min, the contribution of FFA to oxidative metabolism continues to increase from approximately 49% to 61% (Ahlborg et al., 1974).

Exercise-induced changes in fuel flux are regulated by hormonal and neurological responses. Prolonged exercise not only induces a fall in insulin levels (Bang et al., 1990) but also an increase in glucagon, catecholamines, and cortisol concentrations (Christensen et al., 1979; Felig & Wahren, 1979; Wasserman, Spalding, Lacy, et al., 1989; Wasserman, Williams, Lacy, Goldstein, & Cherrington, 1989), leading to enhanced muscle glycogenolysis and the accumulation of glucose-6-phosphate. Although insulin secretion decreases to facilitate hepatic glucose production and lipolysis from adipose tissue, blood insulin concentrations are maintained at a small but adequate level to permit augmented glucose uptake. Glucagon helps maintain glucose homeostasis during exercise by playing a poorly understood role in increasing hepatic glucose production. Epinephrine is believed not only to play a role in enhanced hepatic glucose production, but also to help increase FFA concentrations by stimulating lipolysis (Christensen et al., 1979). Hepatic glucose production may also be influenced by sympathetic innervation of the liver (Jarhult, Anderson, Holst, Moghimzadeh, & Nobin, 1980).

Prolonged exercise results in a greater reduction in insulin levels in the portal as compared to peripheral circulation, indicating that strenuous exercise reduces insulin secretion as well as its removal (Cardin, Doiro, & Lavoie, 1991). Muscle protein synthesis is stimulated in postexercise recovery and muscle mass is usually maintained even though exercise may cause muscle protein breakdown (Carraro, Stuart, Hartl, Rosenblatt, & Wolfe, 1990). Garretto, Richter, Goodman, & Ruderman (1984) reported two phases of postexercise glycogen resynthesis. Phase I is immediately after exercise when muscle glycogen is depleted and glucose utilization is increased, whether insulin is present or not. Phase II is an insulin-dependent phase that occurs 2.5 hr after exercise. Glycogen concentrations are restored and only enhanced insulin sensitivity persists. However, increased glucose uptake can persist for 12 to 16 hr following a single bout of intense exercise (Devlin, Hirshman, Horton, & Horton, 1987; Devlin & Horton, 1985).

Type of Exercise Performed: Insulin Sensitivity

The intensity and duration of acute exercise have both short- and long-term effects on insulin mediated glucose uptake (Mikines, Sonne, Farrell, Tronier, & Galbo, 1988). Incremental high-intensity exercise performed for 12 min by trained athletes resulted in a state of insulin resistance lasting for up to 3 hr (Kjaer, Farrel, Christensen, & Galbo, 1986). Others also have found reduced insulin sensitivity 4 hr after intermittent bouts of exercise performed at 70% of $\dot{V}O_2$max (Devlin, Barlow, & Horton, 1989). In fact, an insulin resistance state has been shown to occur many hours later in those with Type II diabetes following high-intensity, exhaustive exercise (Kjaer et al., 1990). In contrast, lower intensity exercise appears not to induce an insulin resistant state. Mikines et al. (1988) reported that 1 hr of bicycling at an intensity of 64% of $\dot{V}O_2$max enhanced insulin sensitivity 1 hr after exercise. The short-term reduced insulin sensitivity following high-intensity exercise may result from a large increase in exercise-induced sympathoadrenal activity (Sacca, Morrone, Cicala, Corso, & Ungaro, 1980). While high-intensity exercise results in a state of insulin resistance, this condition does not persist; insulin sensitivity has been shown to be enhanced 12 to 16 hr after exhaustive exercise in those with NIDDM (Kjaer et al., 1990).

Plasma glucose concentrations in highly trained athletes as compared with untrained individuals are greater at moderate-intensity to high-intensity effort during acute exercise (Kjaer et al., 1986; Kjaer et al., 1990). Carbohydrate fuels are spared, lipids are utilized at the expense of carbohydrates, and the rate of muscle glycogen breakdown and liver glycogen depletion decreases. Insulin receptor–associated tyrosine kinase activity is not altered following exercise in trained rats (Dohm, Sinha, & Caro, 1987), and increased insulin binding to muscle has not consistently been found (Bonen, Tan, & Watson-Wright, 1984; Treadway, James, Burcel, &

Ruderman, 1989). For these reasons, it has been suggested that enhanced insulin action postexercise may result from postreceptor events (Richter, Turcotte, Hespel, & Kiens, 1992). Ten days after exercise cessation, normal individuals lose exercise-induced improvements in glucose tolerance (Heath et al., 1983). Insulin sensitivity in highly trained athletes, measured by the euglycemic hyperinsulin test, shows a marked reduction within 60 hr following the last bout of exercise (Burstein et al., 1985).

Insulin- and Exercise-Mediated Glucose Uptake

The main tissue involved in insulin-stimulated glucose uptake is skeletal muscle (Baron, Brechtel, Wallace, & Edelman, 1988; DeFronzo et al., 1981). Epinephrine inhibits insulin-mediated glucose uptake, but it has no effect on noninsulin-mediated glucose uptake (Baron, Wallace, & Olefsky, 1987). Noninsulin-mediated glucose uptake pathways in blood cells, splanchnic tissue, and the central and peripheral nervous systems continue glucose uptake in the absence of insulin (Ferrannini et al., 1985). Skeletal muscles can slightly enhance glucose uptake without insulin present by contractile activity, but insulin is required for the full response (Bjorkman, Miles, Wasserman, Lickley, & Franic, 1988). Exercise stimulates increased glucose transport in skeletal muscle. This probably results from greater insulin sensitivity, rather than an attenuation or reversal of the exercise-induced increase in insulin-dependent glucose transport activity (Gulve, Cartee, Zierath, Corpus, & Holloszy, 1990).

Facilitated glucose transport in muscle tissue is effectuated by glucose transporter molecules (James, Strube, & Mueckler, 1989). Figure 4.1 is a schematic representation of distinct membrane fractions isolated from skeletal muscle as reported by Klip et al. (1992). The two major stimulators of glucose transport in skeletal muscle are insulin and repeated muscle contractions (Sternlicht, Barnard, & Grimditch, 1989; Wallberg-Henriksson, 1987). Rodnick, Piper, Slot, and James (1992) have outlined the known family of structurally related proteins that facilitate glucose transport (Glut 1, Glut 2, Glut 3, Glut 4, Glut 5) and their presently known distribution. The isoform Glut 4 is the one primarily distributed in muscle and fat and is the major protein translocated from an intracellular pool to the cell surface in response to insulin (Douen, Ramlal, Rastogi, et al., 1990) and contractile activity of muscle (Douen et al., 1990; King et al., 1989). Exercise has a major stimulator effect to increase the number of glucose transporters at the plasma membrane (Douen et al., 1989; Fushiki, Wells, Tapscott, & Dohm, 1989; Goodyear et al., 1990; King et al., 1989) as well as to increase the activity of the transporters. This response is similar to that of insulin (Klip, Ramlal, Young, & Holloszy, 1987).

The contribution of fuel sources will always depend on exercise intensity and duration (McLellan & Jacobs, 1991; Sahlin, 1990). Other influencing factors are

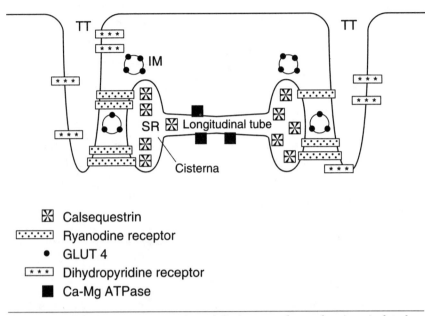

Figure 4.1   Schematic representation of distinct membrane fractions isolated from skeletal muscle. It is proposed that Glut 4 glucose transporters reside largely in an intracellular organelle, hypothetically situated near the transverse tubule (TT) and sarcoplasmic reticulum (SR) cisternae. This organelle would be distinct from TT and cisternae, based on their isolation as a membrane fraction enriched in Glut 4 transporters and devoid of TT and sarcoplasmic reticulum markers. The organelle would furnish the plasma membrane (PM) with glucose transporters in response to insulin. However, a basal amount of glucose transporters is present in the PM of unstimulated muscles (not shown). IM = intracellular membrane.

- the individual's physical fitness level,
- the individual's previous nutritional state,
- the individual's age,
- the type of exercise performed, and
- the existing disease state of the individual (e.g., hyperglycemia, hyperinsulinemia, etc.)

Hyperglycemia, a disease factor associated with the diabetes syndrome, may disrupt the normal sequelae of fuel homeostasis. In people without diabetes, however, hyperglycemia may not have that effect—experimentally induced hyperglycemia in highly trained cyclists did not alter muscle glycogen metabolism during 2 hr of intense cycling (Coyle, Hamilton, Alonso, Montain, & Ivy, 1991).

Cardiopulmonary and Blood Flow Factors

Cardiopulmonary factors greatly change in response to acute exercise. A marked increase in muscle blood flow occurs to adequately supply the contracting muscle's critical needs such as insulin, glucose, oxygen, and other nutrients. A synergistic interaction between exercise and insulin enhances peripheral glucose uptake (DeFronzo, Ferrannini, Sato, Felig, & Wahren, 1981). Increased glucose uptake in skeletal muscle during exercise correlates with increased blood flow—the increased blood flow and increased capillary surface area in working muscle probably account for this synergism. Although increased glucose uptake in skeletal muscle correlates with increased blood flow, it is unlikely that the increased blood flow regulates glucose uptake by the muscle (DeFronzo et al., 1981). Rather, the muscle uptake of glucose is believed to be controlled by the interaction between insulin and epinephrine; insulin and exercise interact synergistically in stimulating total glucose utilization and carbohydrate oxidation (Wasserman et al., 1991). Muscle glycogen depletion during prolonged exercise probably accounts for muscular fatigue (Bergstrom, Hermansen, Hultman, & Saltin, 1967). Hence, changes in insulin, glucagon, and epinephrine are probably relevant to the prevention of hypoglycemia during exercise (Hirsch et al., 1991; Marker et al. 1991).

Postexercise Recovery

The period following acute, strenuous, prolonged exercise is characterized by a change from a catabolic period to an anabolic period. Muscle glycogen stores are replenished for many hours (Maehlum, Felig, & Wahren, 1978), and net protein resynthesis occurs (Millward et al., 1982; Wolfe, Goodenough, Wolfe, Royle, & Nadel, 1982). Splanchnic glucose output in postrecovery may increase by 300%. Ingested glucose during recovery should be used for replenishing muscle glycogen rather than for hepatic glycogen replenishment (Maehlum et al., 1978). The postrecovery increase in glucose uptake is primarily due to an increase in glucose availability (Bourey et al., 1990). Decreased insulin levels occurring during exercise result in enhanced insulin secretion during recovery (Kirwan, Bourey, Kohrt, Staten, & Holloszy, 1991) and may be secondary to exercise-induced increases in endogenous opioids (Farrell, Sonne, Mikines, & Galbo, 1988). Postexercise increases in insulin levels are probably important for replenishing the muscle glycogen stores.

Rates of total glucose disposal remain constant, but glucose metabolic pathways shift from primarily oxidative to nonoxidative during postexercise recovery. Exercise modulates the insulin-induced translocation of glucose transporters, and in the recovery period insulin may alter the intrinsic activity of plasma membrane glucose transporters (Douen, Ramial, Cartee, & Klip, 1990). An increase in both glucose transporter numbers and intrinsic activity following exercise may remain up to 2 hr with the transporter number response lasting longer than the intrinsic activity response.

Increased nonoxidative glucose disposal rate may prolong reduced blood glucose levels. Maehlum et al. (1978) reported that glucose levels may be suppressed following high-intensity exercise for long periods of time—muscle glycogen stores were found to be only 50% replenished in 12 hours. Studies of increased insulin-stimulated glucose uptake that compared active to inactive extremities indicate that postexercise increases in insulin sensitivity involve local, not systemic, factors (Annuzzi, Riccardi, Capaldo, & Kaijser, 1991). Skeletal muscle not directly involved in exercise continued glycogenolysis during the early (40 to 240 min) recovery phases following acute strenuous exercise with the release of lactate and alanine as precursors for gluconeogenesis (Ahlborg & Felig, 1982; Devlin & Horton, 1989).

Type II Diabetes

Metabolic responses to acute exercise may differ in the individual with NIDDM as compared with the healthy individual due to abnormal insulin secretion, tissue insulin sensitivity, and hepatic glucose production associated with the diabetes syndrome. An individual with NIDDM not only has an abnormal insulin secretion response to a glucose stimulus, but also has no inhibition of insulin secretion in response to exercise. Peripheral insulin resistance is present in subjects with NIDDM and is associated with an impairment in insulin binding to insulin receptors and postreceptor abnormalities.

Substrate Utilization in Contracting Muscle

Fuel utilization during exercise is abnormal in the diabetic state. When rats with mild streptozotocin diabetes performed muscular exercise they displayed an abnormal glucose uptake response to insulin (Nesher, Karl, & Kipnis, 1985; Wallberg-Henriksson & Holloszy, 1985) and abnormal lipid mobilization (Koivisto, Akerblom, & Nikkila, 1976; Koivisto, Nikkila, & Akerblom, 1975). Because obesity, hypertension, poor diet, and a lack of routine exercise may exacerbate these abnormalities, acute exercise by people with these conditions may worsen the glycemic control of NIDDM subjects. These factors may alter fuel homeostasis independently or in combination both during and following exercise in the recovery period.

A defect in the glucose transport system of skeletal muscle may be associated with insulin resistance in NIDDM (Andréasson, Galuska,

Thörne, Sonnenfeldt, & Wallberg-Henriksson, 1991; Butler, Kryshak, Marsh, & Rizza, 1990). However, Glut 4 appears to be expressed normally in muscle of people with Type II diabetes, despite marked insulin resistance (Pedersen et al., 1990). Additional research is needed to ascertain if increased expression of Glut 4 in people with NIDDM would enhance insulin-stimulated glucose uptake (Rodnick et al., 1992). Wallberg-Henriksson and Holloszy (1985) have performed elaborate studies using rat epitrochlearis muscle preparation to investigate the regulation of glucose in diabetic skeletal muscle. They demonstrated glucose transport in response to muscle contraction, but the response was markedly attenuated in comparison with the capacity of healthy control muscles. These investigators noted that this reduction in exercise-induced increase in glucose transport of diabetic tissue mirrored the decrease in insulin-stimulated glucose transport. It is generally believed that decreased insulin sensitivity results from defects both at the receptor level (insulin binding) and at the receptor level involving a post-binding step. The latter defect may be secondary to tyrosine kinase activity. Furthermore, a decreased number of glucose transporters or a defect in the translocation mechanism of the transporters may play a role in decreased insulin sensitivity (see Figure 4.2) (Wallberg-Henriksson, 1992).

Acute Exercise and Glycemic Control

Koivisto and DeFronzo (1984) studied glucose homeostasis in 6 middle-aged, regular-weight, hyperglycemic (140 mg/dl), hyperinsulinemic

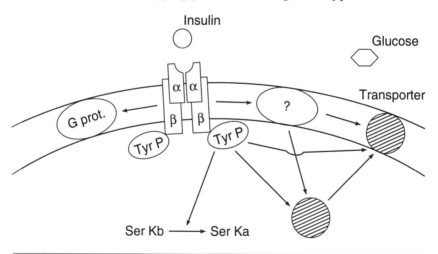

Figure 4.2 Model of insulin action on glucose transport in insulin-sensitive cells. G prot. = G-protein, Tyr P = tyrosine kinase phosphorylation, Ser = serine.
Reprinted with permission from *Diabetes Care,* **15** (Suppl. 4), 1992, p. 1778. Copyright © 1992 by American Diabetes Association, Inc.

(23 μ/ml) Type II diabetics during a 3-hr cycle ergometer test at an intensity of 40% V̇O₂max. A 40 mg/dl drop was noted in elevated plasma basal glucose levels during the acute exercise, a magnitude of response twice that observed in healthy individuals during similar exercise (Koivisto, Hendler, Nadel, & Felig, 1982). Final glucose levels remained higher than normal values even though marked reductions in plasma glucose levels were found in these NIDDM subjects during prolonged exercise. Elevated basal insulin levels decreased to near-normal levels during the 3 hr of exercise, to concentrations comparable to controls, yet plasma glucose concentrations remained high compared with values for nondiabetic individuals. These investigators explained the elevated glucose levels by the presence of insulin resistance in the subjects with NIDDM.

The magnitude of the fall in glucose levels during acute strenuous exercise is closely associated with the duration of exercise. Lower glucose levels at 40 min of exercise as compared with values at 20 min have been reported (Paternostro-Bayles, Wing, & Robertson, 1989). However, variable results have been reported for short durations of exercise, probably due to the intensity of exercise. Short periods of high-intensity exercise markedly lower glycogen stores in active muscles and may be sufficient to lower glucose levels. Schneider et al. (1987) studied the effects of 30 min of cycling at 70% to 75% of V̇O₂max in those with NIDDM. Plasma glucose levels decreased in the NIDDM group but not in lean controls matched for previous activity. Those with NIDDM displayed abnormal glucoregulation and insulin concentrations and did not decrease plasma glucose concentrations as expected with acute exercise.

When Jenkins, Furler, Bruce, and Chisholm (1988) studied regulation of hepatic glucose output during moderate exercise in NIDDM, their results showed a heterogenetic glucose turnover response to moderate exercise. Plasma glucose levels either decreased, showed little change, or increased in different individuals. Hepatic glucose response showed similar heterogenetic results ranging from minimal to a normal response. Mean glucose utilization in NIDDM was also attenuated, but it was not significantly different than in controls. Unlike healthy subjects, subjects with NIDDM had impaired feedback control of hepatic glucose output by circulating plasma glucose during moderate exercise. This varied response may account for why, in another study, a single bout of exercise did not result in improved glucose tolerance in patients with mild NIDDM (Rogers et al., 1988).

Obesity

The combination of heightened plasma insulin and diminished catecholamine response to acute exercise may account in part for subnormal plasma substrate increments that distinguished the obese from the nonobese individual (Gustafson, Farrell, & Kalkhoff, 1990). Whereas plasma insulin levels reportedly decrease during exercise and return to normal by 5-min postexercise, they are much higher in obese individuals than in lean controls (Gustafson et al., 1990). Yale, Leiter, and Marliss (1989) studied the metabolic responses to intense exercise in obese and lean subjects and found that obese individuals had higher resting plasma glucose and insulin levels and elevated blood glycerol concentrations. No changes were seen in plasma glucose or insulin levels during exercise. During the recovery period, both glucose and insulin concentrations were elevated in the obese as compared with lean controls. These results raise the possibility of transient hepatic insulin resistance during postexercise periods, which may be necessary for restoration of depleted muscle glycogen. FFA levels decreased during exercise in both lean and obese subjects. Blood glycerol was higher in the obese subjects than the lean subjects during the postexercise recovery period. Plasma norepinephrine levels increased similarly in both groups and returned immediately to baseline values after exercise. In contrast, plasma epinephrine levels in response to exercise were markedly attenuated in the obese individual. The authors concluded that this study suggests a greater insulin resistance in obese subjects during the recovery period after exercise.

Minuk, Hanna, Marliss, Vranic, and Zinman (1980) studied the effect of acute exercise on glucose metabolism in obese subjects with NIDDM. They found that plasma glucose levels were reduced acutely in obese subjects with NIDDM following 45 min of moderate exercise. The reason for this drop is that hepatic glucose production was less than the increase in muscle glucose uptake during exercise. Whereas exercise reduced glucose levels in this study, glucose levels were still above normal concentrations. A subsequent study from this laboratory examined glucoregulatory and metabolic response to acute exercise in obese subjects with NIDDM (Minuk et al., 1981). These researchers reported that obese NIDDM patients with mild fasting hyperglycemia and normal insulin concentrations on diet therapy alone or on diet therapy in combination with sulfonylurea therapy reduced their blood glucose levels by 35 mg/dl and 37 mg/dl, respectively, during 45 min of exercise at an intensity of 60% $\dot{V}O_2$max. Hepatic glucose production was elevated at rest, and glucose metabolic clearance rate was suppressed in subjects with NIDDM. During exercise, glucose uptake increased normally, but hepatic glucose production was abnormally low, which accounted for the decrease in plasma glucose levels of the NIDDM group. Plasma immunoreactive insulin was elevated at rest and failed to decline normally with exercise. The observed reduction in glucose levels during sustained exercise was presumably due to the fact that insulin secretion was not inhibited in these patients with NIDDM. Changes in insulin binding probably was not a factor because insulin binding to monocytes in obese individuals following exercise has been reported to be diminished (Koivisto, Somna, & Felig, 1980).

Insulin-resistant obese Zucker rats, running at approximately 72% to 73% of their maximal oxygen consumption during an exercise bout, showed significantly higher respiratory exchange ratios as compared with lean control rats (Torgan, Brozinick, Willems, & Ivy, 1990). The obese rats required 54% more carbohydrate utilization during exercise as compared with the lean controls. Fuel utilization by various muscles did not differ between the obese and lean groups. Total liver glycogen values, in contrast, were much higher in the obese rats, and the obese rats used twice as much liver glycogen as their lean counterparts. Obese rats had higher levels of blood glucose and insulin than the lean rats during acute exercise. This study concluded that obese, insulin-resistant rats have a greater dependency on carbohydrates as a substrate during exercise than lean controls, and that the major source of this carbohydrate appears to be liver glycogen. Friedman, Lemon, and Finkelstein (1990) studied the effect of prior exercise and obesity on skeletal muscle uptake of amino acid in the genetically obese Zucker rat. At rest, obese rats displayed lower amino acid uptake than lean controls. Following exercise, both obese and lean animals increased amino acid uptake, with relative greater increases in the obese rats. The authors concluded that lack of exercise may in part contribute to reduced basal skeletal muscle amino acid uptake.

Obese patients and nonobese individuals with NIDDM show decreased insulin binding and reduced receptor tyrosine kinase activity (Caro, Dohm, Pories, & Sinha, 1989; Obermaier-Kusser et al., 1989). In contrast to nonobese Type II diabetics (Pedersen et al., 1990), obese NIDDM patients also demonstrate a decreased number of glucose transporters in their skeletal muscles (Caro et al., 1989; Dohm et al., 1991).

Hormonal Response

Hormonal abnormalities involving insulin metabolism may be especially important during muscle contractions because hormones play a major role in mediating many metabolic responses. Kjaer et al. (1990) studied glucose regulation and hormonal responses to maximal exercise in 7 subjects with NIDDM and 7 nondiabetic subjects. They found that glucose production increased more than glucose utilization did during exercise in both groups of subjects. The increase in glucose production appeared more quickly in NIDDM subjects, but glucose uptake was inhibited compared with controls. Plasma epinephrine and glucose levels in response to exercise were higher in the NIDDM subjects compared with controls. Utilization of the euglycemic clamp technique, at an infusion rate of 40 microcuries per meter per min of insulin with plasma glucose maintained at basal levels, resulted in a higher glucose disposal rate in the NIDDM subjects as compared with controls 24 hr after exercise. The authors concluded that the exaggerated counterregulatory hormone response to exercise resulted in a 60-min period of postexercise hyperglycemia and hyperinsulinemia in the NIDDM individual. An increased insulin effect on glucose production occurred 24 hr after exercise.

Insulin-deprived alloxan diabetic (A-D) dogs were run for 90 min to study the role of glucagon during exercise (Wasserman, Lickley, & Vranic, 1985). A-D dogs, when compared to normal dogs, had similar hepatic glucose production, lower glucose metabolic clearance rates, and higher plasma glucose and FFA levels, both at rest and during exercise. The immunoreactive glucagon of the A-D dogs was higher at rest and increased at a threefold greater rate than in controls during exercise. Immunoreactive insulin levels were lower by 68% at rest in the A-D dogs, levels similar to those of controls during exercise. A-D dogs, as compared with normal dogs, had similar blood concentrations of epinephrine, norepinephrine, cortisol, and lactate at rest. A-D dogs had greater increments of norepinephrine, cortisol, and lactate during exercise. Suppression of glucagon by somatostatin in A-D dogs resulted in markedly reduced hepatic glucose production during exercise, in turn resulting in a large reduction in plasma glucose levels and reduced glucose uptake. Because glucose levels never reached the hypoglycemia range, excessive counterregulation did not occur in the A-D dogs.

Muscle Enzymes

The rate-limiting enzyme for glycogen synthesis, glycogen synthase, appears to be normally activated during high-intensity acute exercise in subjects with NIDDM (Devlin et al., 1987). Because insulin-mediated nonoxidative glucose uptake increases after glycogen-depleting exercise and glycogen synthase activity remains normal, individuals with Type II diabetes probably have a defect in glucose transport (Devlin, 1992). Support for this contention comes from reports showing that in disease states such as NIDDM insulin-stimulated glucose transport in skeletal muscle is impaired (Dohm et al., 1988).

Cardiorespiratory

Cardiorespiratory demands in response to acute exercise are more likely to be abnormal in individuals with NIDDM due to their higher risk for advanced atherosclerotic cardiovascular disease. The atherogenic risk factors may be present for years—they have been demonstrated in prediabetic subjects (Haffner, Stern, Hazuda, Mitchel, & Paterson, 1990)—and cause the development of major vascular intimal lesions long before NIDDM is detected. The postexercise period, when the anabolic response to acute exercise is occurring, may be of clinical importance because this may be the time when metabolism is normalized.

Postexercise

Devlin and Horton (1989) showed that an anabolic state exists for a long period following acute intense exercise. They studied metabolic fuel utilization during postexercise recovery in lean normal, obese, and NIDDM subjects. Rates of total glucose disposal increased only in the obese and NIDDM subjects, but the rates did not reach normal levels (Table 4.1). Both early (0 to 4 hr) and late (12 to 16 hr) periods following intense exercise were characterized by a shift to lower glucose oxidation and an increased rate of nonoxidative glucose disposal in all subjects when compared to preexercise measures. Vastus lateralis muscle glycogen synthase activities increased similarly in all subjects, demonstrating increased glycogen resynthesis following acute exercise. This response correlated to an increased rate of nonoxidative glucose disposal (Figure 4.3). Results of the insulin suppression tests used in this study showed that endogenous glucose production was not totally suppressed in the obese subjects, either before or after exercise.

Insulin Binding, Insulin Sensitivity, and Thermic Effect of Insulin

A single bout of high-intensity exercise has been shown to improve peripheral and hepatic insulin sensitivity in subjects with NIDDM (Devlin et al., 1987; Heath et al., 1983). Koivisto, Soman, DeFronzo, and Felig (1980) examined insulin binding to monocytes in highly trained long-distance runners and in sedentary controls at rest and after exercising at 40% of maximal aerobic power on a cycle ergometer for 3 hours. The runners, as compared with controls, displayed a 69% greater insulin binding to monocytes at rest due to an increase in binding capacity rather than binding affinity. Acute exercise resulted in a 31% decrease in insulin binding in the runners. In contrast, a 35% rise in insulin binding was observed in the controls. These investigators suggested that the reduction in insulin binding during acute exercise found in runners, as compared with controls, may contribute to increased fat utilization and a shift from carbohydrate utilization in trained individuals. Obesity may alter insulin binding, both at rest and during acute exercise. Koivisto et al. (1980) studied insulin binding in obese and nonobese subjects before and during 3 hr of stationary cycling. At basal conditions, obese subjects showed a 25% lower insulin binding to monocytes as compared with controls. Insulin

Table 4.1   Metabolic Fuel Utilization During Postexercise Recovery

Measure	Lean	Obese	NIDDM
Total glucose disposal	No change	Increase	Increase
Glucose oxidation	Decrease	Decrease	Decrease
Nonoxidative glucose disposal	Increase	Increase	Increase
Muscle glycogen synthase activity	Normal	Normal	Normal
Endogenous glucose production rate	No change	Resistance	Decrease

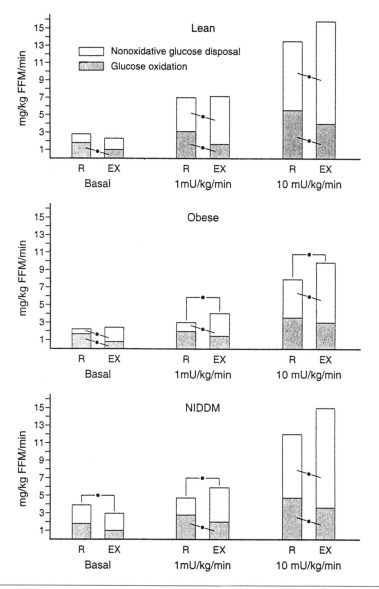

Figure 4.3 Glucose disposal rates (mg · kg fat-free mass^{-1} [FFM] · min^{-1}) without (R) and with (Ex) prior exercise in the basal state and during the steady-state periods of the 40 mU · m^{-2} · min^{-1} (low dose) and 400 mU · m^{-2} · min^{-1} (high dose) insulin infusions, in lean, obese, and NIDDM humans. Dot (•) indicates significant differences (P < 0.05) in total glucose disposal (top of bars), nonoxidative glucose disposal (side of bars, upper), and glucose oxidation (side of bars, lower), comparing the postexercised (Ex) with the nonexercised (R) state.

Reprinted with permission from *Diabetes Care*, **15** (Suppl. 4), 1992, p. 1692. Copyright © by American Diabetes Association, Inc.

binding to monocytes increased minimally in the obese group (13%) as compared with controls (36%), indicating that obesity diminishes this response to acute exercise. Koivisto and Yki-Jarvinen (1987) studied insulin binding and the rate of glucose transport in adipocytes of normal controls at rest and after 3 hr of exercise on a cycle ergometer. Insulin binding to adipocytes showed no change, plasma glucose and insulin levels decreased, and serum free fatty acid concentrations increased with acute exercise. Insulin binding to adipocytes was unaltered, the rate of basal glucose transport clearance decreased, and the insulin-stimulated glucose transport increased. Because acute exercise did not result in an increase in binding to adipocytes as shown for blood cells, these investigators concluded that insulin binding appears to be tissue-specific and may not always parallel changes in glucose transport.

Strenuous exercise resulting in muscle glycogen depletion can alter insulin metabolism as well. Krotkiewski and Gorski (1986) found that plasma insulin C-peptide concentrations during acute exercise were reduced both in control and obese individuals with Type II diabetes. Whereas plasma insulin levels returned to normal quickly in the control group, higher values were found during recovery in the obese Type II group. Molar ratios of plasma C-peptide to insulin for this group were more attenuated during the 15-min recovery period, but they returned to normal within the next 15 min. This suggested to the investigators that reduced insulin removal in the obese NIDDM subjects may have been a major contributing factor to the increase of plasma insulin concentrations observed during recovery.

Burstein, Epstein, Shapiro, Charuzi, and Karnielli (1990) studied the effect of acute exercise on the action of insulin to stimulate glucose disposal in 6 obese NIDDM subjects, 7 obese normoglycemic subjects, and 6 lean healthy controls. In the basal state, the metabolic clearance rate of glucose was reduced in the obese subjects as compared with lean controls. Exercise resulted in an increased metabolic clearance rate of glucose for both obese NIDDM and obese normoglycemic subjects, but not in the lean controls. Although the metabolic clearance rate was enhanced by acute exercise, it remained below normal. Results suggest an improvement in peripheral insulin sensitivity following acute exercise but not to normal levels (see Figure 4.3 on p. 99).

Devlin and Horton (1989) studied fuel utilization postexercise in lean, obese, and NIDDM subjects. In all groups, prior high-intensity exercise decreased glucose oxidation and enhanced nonoxidative glucose disposal as a result of resynthesis of depleted muscle glycogen. Obese and NIDDM subjects displayed increased total rates of glucose disposal following acute exercise. This finding suggested amelioration of the postreceptor defects in insulin action as a part of the diabetic syndrome in insulin-resistant subjects. Interestingly, Devlin and Horton (1989) showed that this occurred for up to 2 hr after high-intensity exercise in subjects with NIDDM. Another important finding was that hepatic insulin sensitivity improved during postexercise recovery in the NIDDM subjects. This is of major interest because postabsorptive rates of hepatic glucose production are higher in individuals with NIDDM and result in elevated glucose levels (DeFronzo, Ferrannini, & Koivisto, 1983). Muscle not involved in exercise may play an important role during postexercise recovery by supplying adequate lactate for gluconeogenesis to replenish glycogen stores in exercised muscle (Ahlborg & Felig, 1982).

Devlin et al. (1987) conducted elaborate metabolic studies to investigate the effect of high-intensity (85% $\dot{V}O_2$max) acute exercise on peripheral and splanchnic insulin sensitivity in obese NIDDM men by measuring rates of total glucose utilization, glucose oxidation, nonoxidative glucose disposal, glucose metabolic clearance rate, and hepatic glucose production after a single bout of high-intensity exercise. The researchers used the insulin clamp technique to determine the effects at two insulin levels. Twelve hours following an acute bout of glycogen-depleting exercise, total glucose disposal was significantly increased at the lower infusion rate, but not at the higher infusion rates as compared with resting values. Devlin and associates concluded that the increase in insulin-stimulated glycogen disposal rate was the result of higher nonoxidative glucose disposal, presumably for glycogen resynthesis. The individuals with NIDDM in this study, as compared with lean subjects without diabetes, displayed a reduced metabolic clearance of glucose during both insulin infusion rates, but it was similar to those found for the obese individuals without diabetes. The basal endogenous glucose reproduction rate was significantly reduced the day following exercise, and this finding was associated with significant reductions of fasting plasma glucose in the obese men with NIDDM.

Devlin and Horton (1986) studied the effect of prior exercise on total energy expenditure and the thermic effect of insulin in obese insulin-resistant people, people with NIDDM, and normal controls. Only the normal controls showed a marked increase in total energy expenditure 12 to 16 hr after exercise. All groups showed decreased glucose and increased lipid oxidation. Obese subjects showed no response in the thermic effect of insulin during low-dose insulin infusion, whereas prior exercise potentiated this response in individuals with NIDDM and controls. Both the NIDDM and control groups responded similarly during high-dose insulin infusion, whereas the obese group displayed an attenuated response. A positive correlation was found between the thermic effect of insulin and insulin-stimulated rates of glucose uptake.

Diabetes and Cardiovascular Response to Acute Exercise

The cardiovascular system is made up of several components, one or many of which may be affected by an altered metabolic or physiologic state. Diabetes may influence the cardiovascular system in a variety of ways. This section will highlight the main effects that Type II diabetes has on the cardiovascular system.

Left Ventricular Function

Mustonen et al. (1988), using equilibrium radionuclide angiocardiography, compared left ventricular systolic function during exercise in middle-aged IDDM and NIDDM subjects without clinical evidence of cardiovascular disease. An increase of less than 5% or a decrease in left ventricular function was observed with exercise in 8 men with IDDM and in 10 men with NIDDM. The metabolic control of glycemia was not related to abnormal left ventricular ejection fractions. These results demonstrate that left ventricular function can be markedly altered in Type II diabetes, even though there are no overt clinical signs of cardiac impairment. Other researchers (Takahashi, Iwasaki, Sugiura, Hasegawa, Tarumi, Matsutani, et al., 1991) studied middle-aged NIDDM patients without clinical evidence of cardiovascular disease to determine the effect of microangiopathic complications and autonomic dysfunction on cardiac function during exercise. None of the subjects had ischemic ST-T segment changes or angina during maximal treadmill exercise testing. No differences were found in left ventricular ejection time (LVET) and preejection periods (PEP) at rest. But LVET was prolonged with a nearly identical PEP response during acute exercise in patients with retinopathy. The results suggested that patients with retinopathy rely on an enhanced ventricular filling in maintaining adequate stroke volume during exercise. Additional work from this laboratory (Takahashi, Iwasaka, Sugiura, Hasegawa, Tarumi, & Inada, 1991) used acute exercise to study the effect of microangiopathic complications and autonomic dysfunction on diastolic time in 19 patients with Type II diabetes. Neither ischemic ST-T segment responses nor chest discomfort was noted during maximal treadmill exercise. Results showed that people with Type II diabetes and retinopathy may be at increased risk for left ventricular dysfunction through diminished subendocardial blood flow as a result of microangiopathy.

Coronary Heart Disease

The prevalence of exercise-induced positive ST-T segment depression has been shown to be similar in 142 asymptomatic Japanese NIDDM patients when compared with 149 nondiabetic control subjects matched for age and sex (Naka et al., 1992). NIDDM subjects with positive treadmill test results, however, had a prevalence of angiographically determined coronary artery stenosis 2.2 times higher than nondiabetic controls with exercise induced ST-T segment changes. Furthermore, diabetic subjects on insulin therapy had a prevalence of silent myocardial ischemia 2.6 times higher than those diabetics not on insulin therapy. Silent myocardial ischemia was 2.5 times higher in diabetic patients with retinopathy. These results are not surprising because NIDDM is associated with both microvascular and macrovascular complications. Hyperinsulinemia may be a major contributing factor to cardiovascular abnormalities by virtue of its metabolic effect on the intima and its contribution to hyperlidemia and hypertension, whereas insulin treatment is usually indicated for poor glycemic control. Impaired fibrinolytic response to exercise has been reported in individuals with Type II diabetes compared with normal controls (Schneider, Kim, Khachadurian, & Ruderman, 1988). Resting levels of plasma fibrinogen, prothrombin time maximal velocity, and activated thromboplastin time were increased postexercise. Activation of fibrinolysis occurred in both groups after exercise, but peak activity and magnitude of response were lower in those with NIDDM. These abnormalities have been suggested as contributing factors to atherogenic vascular disease.

Callaham et al. (1989) retrospectively studied 1,747 subjects to determine the prognosis of silent ischemia in an unselected group of patients referred for exercise testing. A major aim was to determine whether age or the presence of myocardial infarction or diabetes mellitus influenced the prevalence of silent myocardial ischemia during acute exercise. Results showed that those with abnormal ST-T segment depression had a greater mortality rate. The prevalence of silent myocardial ischemia during exercise testing was not significantly different among patients with recent, past, or no myocardial infarction or with insulin-dependent or non-insulin-dependent diabetes mellitus.

Cardiac Metabolism

Donckier et al. (1989) studied atrial natriuretic factor release during exercise in three groups of individuals matched for age and sex, including normal healthy subjects, 7 diabetic patients with cardiac autonomic neuropathy, and 7 diabetic patients without cardiac autonomic neuropathy. Plasma atrial natriuretic factor increased threefold in all three groups. The chronotropic response to exercise was blunted in both diabetic groups but to a greater degree in those with cardiac autonomic neuropathy. Results showed that autonomic activation plays a major role in atrial natriuretic factor release during exercise in both healthy subjects and those with diabetes, whether they had cardiac autonomic neuropathy or not. Because patients without cardiac autonomic neuropathy displayed impaired chronotropic responses to exercise, researchers suggested that early damages of autonomic function appear to be present in patients who aren't demonstrating cardiac autonomic neuropathy.

Blood Pressure

Eleven normotensive, sedentary subjects with NIDDM displayed greater systolic blood pressure values in response to a steady exercise level of 70 to 75 watts on the bicycle ergometer than 11 controls (Blake, Levin, & Koyal, 1990). Systolic blood pressures were 208 ± 6.0 versus 177 ± 3.0 mm of mercury, respectively, for NIDDM and nondiabetic subjects of comparable age and body mass. Heart rate responses and diastolic blood pressure responses to mild exercise did not differ between the NIDDM and control groups during acute exercise.

Romanelli et al. (1989) have shown that microalbuminuria induced by exercise in hypertensive IDDM and NIDDM subjects with stage II nephropathy is blunted better by an angiotensin-converting enzyme inhibitor than by a calcium channel blocker.

Summary

Enhanced hepatic insulin sensitivity resulting from acute exercise may improve hyperglycemia in individuals with NIDDM. Substrate utilization during the postexercise recovery period appears to favorably influence glucose homeostasis in subjects with Type II diabetes and to relate to an increase in nonoxidative glucose disposal, presumably due to an increased muscle glycogen synthesis rate. Routine bouts of exercise (exercise training), therefore, may help maintain euglycemia in subjects with NIDDM. With careful assessment, the cardiovascular benefits of regular exercise may prove beneficial in preventing or forestalling deterioration of the cardiovascular system in NIDDM.

The overall state of health and the metabolic environment are important in determining the individual's response to acute exercise. Administering oral hypoglycemic agents and the specifics of medical treatment need careful attention when planning exercise for patients with Type II diabetes. The cumulative effects of repeated exercise sessions and regular exercise will be discussed in chapter 5.

References

Ahlborg, G., & Felig, P. (1982). Lactate and glucose exchange across the forearm, legs, and splanchnic bed during and after prolonged leg exercise. *Journal of Clinical Investigation, 69*(1), 45-54.

Ahlborg, G., Felig, P., Hagenfeldt, L., Hendler, R., & Wahren, J. (1974). Substrate turnover during prolonged exercise in man: Splanchnic and leg metabolism of glucose, free fatty acids and amino acids. *Journal of Clinical Investigation, 53*, 1078-1084.

Andréasson, K., Galuska, D., Thörne, A., Sonnenfeldt, T., & Wallberg-Henriksson, H. (1991). Decreased insulin-stimulated 3-O-methylglucose transport in *in vitro* incubated muscle strips from Type II diabetic patients. *Acta Physiologica Scandinavica, 142*, 255-260.

Annuzzi, G., Riccardi, G., Capaldo, B., & Kaijser, L. (1991). Increased insulin-stimulated glucose uptake by exercised human muscles one day after prolonged physical exercise. *European Journal of Clinical Investigation, 21*(1), 6-12.

Bang, P., Brandt, J., Degerblad, M., Enberg, G., Kaijser, L., Thoren, M., & Hall, K. (1990). Exercise-induced changes in insulin-like growth factors and their low molecular weight binding protein in healthy subjects and patients with growth hormone deficiency. *European Journal of Clinical Investigation, 21*(1), 6-12.

Baron, A.D., Brechtel, G., Wallace, P., & Edelman, S.V. (1988). Rates and tissue sites of noninsulin- and insulin-mediated glucose uptake in humans. *American Journal of Physiology, 255,* E769-E774.

Baron, A.D., Wallace, P., & Olefsky, J.M. (1987). In vivo regulation of non-insulin-mediated and insulin-mediated glucose uptake by epinephrine. *Journal of Clinical Endocrinology Metabolism, 65*(5), 889-895.

Bergstrom, J., Hermansen, L., Hultman, E., & Saltin, B. (1967). Diet, muscle glycogen and physical performance. *Acta Physiologica Scandinavica, 71*(2), 140-150.

Bjorkman, O., Miles, P., Wasserman, D., Lickley, L., & Vranic, M. (1988). Regulation of glucose turnover during exercise in pancreatectomized, totally insulin-deficient dogs. Effects of beta-adrenergic blockade. *Journal of Clinical Investigation, 81*(6), 1759-1767.

Blake, G.A., Levin, S.R., & Koyal, S.N. (1990). Exercise-induced hypertension in normotensive patients with NIDDM. *Diabetes Care, 13*(7), 799-801.

Bonen, A., Tan, M.H., & Watson-Wright, W.M. (1984). Effects of exercise on insulin binding and glucose metabolism in muscle. *Canadian Journal of Physiology and Pharmacology, 62,* 1500-1504.

Bourey, R.E., Coggan, A.R., Kohrt, W.M., Kirwan, J.P., King, D.S., & Holloszy, J.O. (1990). Effect of exercise on glucose disposal: Response to a maximal insulin stimulus. *Journal of Applied Physiology, 69*(1), 299-304.

Burstein, R., Epstein, Y., Shapiro, Y., Charuzi, I., & Karnielli, E. (1990). Effect of an acute bout of exercise on glucose disposal in human obesity. *Journal of Applied Physiology, 69*(1), 299-304.

Burstein, R., Polychronakos, C., Toews, C.J., MacDougall, J.D., Guyda, H.J., & Posner, B.I. (1985). Acute reversal of the enhanced insulin action in trained athletes. *Diabetes, 34,* 756-760.

Butler, P.C., Kryshale, E.J., Schwenk, W.F., Haymond, M.W., & Rizza, R.A. (1990). Hepatic and extrahepatic responses to insulin in NIDDM and nondiabetic humans. Assessment in absence of artifact introduced by tritiated nonglucose contaminants. *Diabetes, 39,* 217-225.

Callaham, P.R., Froelicher, V.F., Klein, J., Risch, M., Dubach, P., & Friis, R. (1989). Exercise-induced silent ischemia: Age, diabetes mellitus, previous myocardial infarction and prognosis. *Journal of American College of Cardiology, 14*(5), 1175-1180.

Cardin, S., Doiron, B., & Lavoie, J.M. (1991). Effect of prolonged exercise on insulin level in the portal and peripheral venous circulation in rats. *International Journal of Sports Medicine, 12*(2), 187-189.

Caro, J.F., Dohm, L.G., Pories, W.J., & Sinha, M.K. (1989). Cellular alterations in liver, skeletal muscle, and adipose tissue responsible for insulin resistance in obesity and Type II diabetes. *Diabetes and Metabolism Review, 5,* 665-689.

Carraro, F., Stuart, C.A., Hartl, W.H., Rosenblatt, J., & Wolfe, R.R. (1990). Effect of exercise and recovery on muscle protein synthesis in human subjects. *American Journal of Physiology, 259*(4 Pt 1), E470-E476.

Christensen, N.J.M., Galbo, H., Hansen, J., Hesse, B., Richter, E.A., & Trap-Jensen, J. (1979). Catecholamines and exercise. *Diabetes, 28*(Suppl. 1), 58-62.

Coggan, A.R. (1991). Plasma glucose metabolism during exercise in humans. *Sports Medicine, 11*(2), 102-124.

Coyle, E.F., Hamilton, M.T., Alonso, J.G., Montain, S.J., & Ivy, J.L. (1991). Carbohydrate metabolism during intense exercise when hyperglycemic. *Journal of Applied Physiology, 70*(2), 834-840.

DeFronzo, R.A., Ferrannini, E., & Koivisto, V. (1983). New concepts in the pathogenesis and treatment of non-insulin-dependent diabetes mellitus. *American Journal of Medicine, 1774*(1A), 52-81.

DeFronzo, R.A., Ferrannini, E., Sato, Y., Felig, P., & Wahren, J. (1981). Synergistic interaction between exercise and insulin on peripheral glucose uptake. *Journal of Clinical Investigation, 68*(6), 1468-1474.

DeFronzo, R.A., Jacot, E., Jequier, E., Maeder, E., Wahren, H., & Felber, J.P. (1981). The effect of insulin on the disposal of intravenous glucose: Results from indirect calorimetry and hepatic and femoral venous catheterization. *Diabetes, 30,* 1000-1007.

Devlin, J.T. (1992). Effects of exercise on insulin sensitivity in humans. *Diabetes Care, 15*(Suppl. 4), 1690-1693.

Devlin, J.T., Barlow, J., & Horton, E.S. (1989). Whole body and regional fuel metabolism during early postexercise recovery. *American Journal of Physiology, 256,* E167-E172.

Devlin, J.T., Hirshman, M., Horton, E.D., & Horton, E.S. (1987). Enhanced peripheral and splanchnic insulin sensitivity in NIDDM men after single bout of exercise. *Diabetes, 36*(4), 434-439.

Devlin, J.T., & Horton, E.S. (1985). Effects of prior high-intensity exercise on glucose metabolism in normal and insulin-resistant men. *Diabetes, 34,* 973-979.

Devlin, J.T., & Horton, E.S. (1986). Potentiation of the thermic effect of insulin by exercise: Differences between lean, obese, and non-insulin-dependent diabetic men. *American Journal of Clinical Nutrition, 43*(6), 884-890.

Devlin, J.T., & Horton, E.S. (1989). Metabolic fuel utilization during post-exercise recovery. *American Journal of Clinical Nutrition, 49,* 944-948.

Dohm, G.L., Elton, C.W., Friedman, J.E., Pilch, P.F., Pories, W.J., Atkinson, S.M., Jr., & Caro, J.F. (1991). Decreased expression of glucose transporter in muscle from insulin-resistant patients. *American Journal of Physiology*, **260**(Endocrinol. Metab. 23), E459-E463.

Dohm, G.L., Sinha, M.K., & Caro, J.F. (1987). Insulin receptor binding and protein kinase activity in muscles of trained rats. *American Journal of Physiology*, **252**, E170-E175.

Dohm, G.L., Tapscott, E.B., Pories, W.J., Dabbs, D.J., Flinkinger, E.G., Meelheim, D., Fushiki, T., Atkinson, S.M., Elton, C.W., & Caro, J. (1988). An in vitro human muscle preparation suitable for metabolic studies. Decreased insulin stimulation of glucose transport in muscle from morbidly obese and diabetic subjects. *Journal of Clinical Investigation*, **82**, 486-494.

Donckier, J.E., DeCoster, P.M., Buysschaert, M., Pieters, D.P., Cauwe, F.M., Robert, A., Brichant, C.M., Berbinschi, A.C., & Ketelslegers, J.M. (1989). Exercise and posture-related changes of atrial natriuretic factor and cardiac function in diabetes. *Diabetes Care*, **12**(7), 475-480.

Douen, A.G., Ramlal, T., Cartee, G.D., & Klip, A. (1990). Exercise modulates the insulin-induced translocation of glucose transporters in rat skeletal muscle. *Federation of European Biochemical Societies Letters*, **26:261**(2), 256-260.

Douen, A.G., Ramlal, T., Klip, A., Young, D.A., Cartee, G.D., & Holloszy, J.O. (1989). Exercise-induced increase in glucose transporters in plasma membranes of rat skeletal muscle. *Endocrinology*, **124**, 449-454.

Douen, A.G., Ramlal, T., Rastogi, S., Bilan, P.J., Cartee, G.D., Vranic, M., Holloszy, J.O., & Klip, A. (1990). Exercise induces recruitment of the "insulin-responsive glucose transporter." Evidence for distinct intracellular insulin- and exercise-recruitable transporter pools in skeletal muscle. *Journal of Biological Chemistry*, **15:265**(23), 13427-13430.

Farrell, P.A., Sonne, B., Mikines, K., & Galbo, H. (1988). Stimulatory role for endogenous opioid peptides on postexercise insulin secretion in rats. *Journal of Applied Physiology*, **65**(2), 744-749.

Felig, P., & Wahren, J. (1979). Role of insulin and glucagon in the regulation of hepatic glucose production during exercise. *Diabetes*, **28**, 71-75.

Ferrannini, E., Smith, J.D., Cobelli, C., Toffolo, G., Pilo, A., & DeFronzo, R.A. (1985). Effects of insulin on the distribution and disposition of glucose in man. *Journal of Clinical Investigation*, **76**(1), 357-364.

Franz, M.J. (1987). Exercise and the management of diabetes mellitus. *Journal of American Diet Association*, **87**(7), 872-880.

Friedman, J.E., Lemon, P.W., & Finkelstein, J.A. (1990). Effects of exercise and obesity on skeletal muscle amino acid uptake. *Journal of Applied Physiology*, **69**(4), 1347-1352.

Fushiki, T., Wells, J.A., Tapscott, E.B., & Dohm, G.L. (1989). Changes in glucose transporters in muscle in response to exercise. *American Journal of Physiology*, **256**, E580-E587.

Garretto, L., Richter, E.A., Goodman, M.N., & Ruderman, N.B. (1984). Enhanced muscle glucose metabolism after exercise in the rat: The two phases. *American Journal of Physiology, 246*, E471-E475.

Gollnick, P.D. (1985). Metabolism of substrates: Energy substrate metabolism during exercise and as modified by training. *Federation Proceedings, 44*, 353-357.

Goodyear, L.J., Hirshman, M.F., King, P.A., Horton, E.D., Thompson, C.M., & Horton, E.S. (1990). Skeletal muscle plasma membrane glucose transport and glucose transporters after exercise. *Journal of Applied Physiology, 68*(1), 193-198.

Gulve, E.A., Cartee, G.D., Zierath, J.R., Corpus, V.M., & Holloszy, J.O. (1990). Reversal of enhanced muscle glucose transport after exercise: Roles of insulin and glucose. *American Journal of Physiology, 259*(5 Pt. 1), E685-E691.

Gustafson, A.B., Farrell, P.A., & Kalkhoff, R.K. (1990). Impaired plasma catecholamine response to submaximal treadmill exercise in obese women. *Metabolism, 39*(4), 10-17.

Haffner, S.M., Stern, M.P., Hazuda, H.P., Mitchel, B.D., & Patterson, J.K. (1990). Cardiovascular risk factors in confirmed prediabetic individuals: Does the clock for coronary heart disease start ticking before the onset of clinical diabetes? *Journal of the American Medical Association, 263*(21), 2893-2898.

Hagenfeldt, L., & Wahren, J. (1968). Human forearm muscle metabolism during exercise. I. Circulatory adaptation to prolonged forearm exercise. *Scandinavian Journal of Clinical and Laboratory Investigation, 21*, 257-262.

Hagenfeldt, L., Wahren, J., Pernow, B., & Raf, L. (1972). Uptake of individual free fatty acids by skeletal muscle and liver in man. *Clinical Investigation, 51*(9), 2324-2330.

Heath, G.W., Gavin, J.R., Hinderliter, J.M., Hagberg, J.M., Bloomfield, S.A., & Holloszy, J.O. (1983). Effects of exercise and lack of exercise on glucose tolerance and insulin sensitivity. *Journal of Applied Physiology, 55*, 512-517.

Henriksson, J. (1977). Training induced adaptation of skeletal muscle and metabolism during submaximal exercise. *Journal of Physiology, 270*, 661-675.

Hermansen, L., Hultman, E., & Saltin, B. (1967). Muscle glycogen during prolonged severe exercise. *Acta Physiologica Scandinavica, 71*, 129-139.

Hirsch, I.B., Marker, J.C., Smith, L.J., Spina, R.J., Parvin, C.A., Holloszy, J.O., & Cryer, P.E. (1991). Insulin and glucagon in prevention of hypoglycemia during exercise in humans. *American Journal of Physiology, 260*(5 Pt. 1), E695-E704.

James, D.E., Strube, M., & Mueckler, M. (1989). Molecular cloning and characterization of an insulin-regulatable glucose transporter. *Nature (Lond.), 338*, 83-87.

Jarhult, J., Anderson, P.O., Holst, J., Moghimzadeh, E., & Nobin, A. (1980). On the sympathetic innervation of the cat's liver and its role for hepatic glucose release. *Acta Physiologica Scandinavica, 110*, 5-11.

Jenkins, A.B., Furler, S.M., Bruce, D.G., & Chisholm, D.J. (1988). Regulation of hepatic glucose output during moderate exercise in non-insulin-dependent diabetes. *Metabolism, 37*(10), 966-972.

Katz, A., Sahlin, K., & Broberg, S. (1991). Regulation of glucose utilization in human skeletal muscle during moderate dynamic exercise. *American Journal of Physiology, 260*(3 Pt. 1), E411-E415.

King, P.A., Hirshman, M.F., Horton, E.D., & Horton, E.D. (1989). Glucose transport in skeletal muscle membrane vesicles from control and exercise rats. *American Journal of Physiology, 257*, C1128-C1134.

Kirwan, J.P., Bourey, R.E., Kohrt, W.M., Staten, M.A., & Holloszy, J.O. (1991). Effects of treadmill exercise to exhaustion on the insulin response to hyperglycemia in untrained men. *Journal of Applied Physiology, 70*(1), 246-250.

Kjaer, M., Farrel, P.A., Christensen, N.J., & Galbo, H. (1986). Increased epinephrine response and inaccurate glucoregulation in exercising athletes. *Journal of Applied Physiology, 61*, 1693-1700.

Kjaer, M., Hollenbeck, C.B., Frey-Hewitt, B., Galbo, H., Haskell, W., & Reaven, G.M. (1990). Glucoregulation and hormonal responses to maximal exercise in non-insulin-dependent diabetes. *Journal of Applied Physiology, 68*(5), 2067-2074.

Klip, A., Marette, A., Dimitrakoudis, D., Ramlal, T., Giacca, A., Shi, Z.Q., & Vranic, M. (1992). Effect of diabetes on glucoregulation: From glucose transporters to glucose metabolism in vivo. *Diabetes Care, 15*(4), 1747-1766.

Klip, A., Ramlal, T., Young, D., & Holloszy, J.O. (1987). Insulin-induced translocation of glucose transporters in rat hindlimb muscles. *FEBS Letters, 224*, 224-230.

Koivisto, V.A., Akerblom, H.K., & Nikkila, A. (1976). Metabolic and hormonal effects of exercise in mild streptozotocin diabetes. *Scandinavian Journal of Clinical Laboratory Investigation, 36*(1), 45-49.

Koivisto, V.A., & DeFronzo, R.A. (1984). Exercise in the treatment of Type II diabetes. *Acta Endocrinologica, 262*(Suppl.), 107-111.

Koivisto, V., Hendler, R., Nadel, E., & Felig, P. (1982). Influence of physical training on the fuel-hormone response to prolonged low intensity exercise. *Metabolism, 31*, 192-197.

Koivisto, V.A., Nikkila, E.A., & Akerblom, H.K. (1975). Influence of norepinephrine and exercise on lipolysis in adipose tissue of diabetic rats. *Diabetologia, 11*(5), 401-405.

Koivisto, V.A., Soman, V.R., DeFronzo, R., & Felig, P. (1980). Effects of acute exercise and training on insulin binding to monocytes and insulin sensitivity in vivo. *Acta Paediatria Scandinavian Supplement, 283*, 70-78.

Koivisto, V.A., Soman, V.R., & Felig, P. (1980). Effects of acute exercise on insulin binding to monocytes in obesity. *Metabolism, 29*(2), 168-172.

Koivisto, V.A., & Yki-Jarvinen, H.J. (1987). Effect of exercise on insulin binding and glucose transport in adipocytes of normal humans. *Journal of Applied Physiology, 63*, 1319-1323.

Krotkiewski, M., & Gorski, J. (1986). Effect of muscular exercise on plasma C-peptide and insulin in obese non-diabetics and diabetics, Type II. *Clinical Physiology, 6*(6), 499-506.

Lindinger, M.I., Heigenhauser, G.J., McKelvie, R.S., & Jones, N.L. (1990). Role of nonworking muscle on blood metabolites and ions with intense intermittent exercise. *American Journal of Physiology, 258*(6 Pt. 2), R1486-R1494.

Maehlum, S., Felig, P., & Wahren, J. (1978). Splanchnic glucose and muscle glycogen metabolism after glucose feeding during postexercise recovery. *American Journal of Physiology, 235*(5), E255-E260.

Maehlum, S., & Hermansen, L. (1978). Muscle glycogen concentration during recovery after prolonged severe exercise in fasting subjects. *Scandinavian Journal of Clinical Laboratory Investigation, 38*(6), 557-560.

Marker, J.C., Hirsch, I.B., Smith, L.J., Parvin, C.A., Holloszy, J.O., & Cryer, P.E. (1991). Catecholamines in prevention of hypoglycemia during exercise in humans. *American Journal of Physiology, 260*(5 Pt 1), E705-E712.

McLellan, T.M., & Jacobs, I. (1991). Muscle glycogen utilization and the expression of relative exercise intensity. *International Journal of Sports Medicine, 12*(1), 21-26.

Mikines, K.J., Sonne, B., Farrell, P.A., Tronier, B., & Galbo, H. (1988). Effect of physical exercise on sensitivity and responsiveness to insulin in man. *American Journal of Physiology, 254*, E248-E259.

Millward, D.J., Davies, C.T., Halliday, D., Wolman, S.L., Matthews, D., & Rennie, M. (1982). Effect of exercise on protein metabolism in humans as explored with stable isotopes. *Federation Procedures, 41*(10), 2686-2691.

Minuk, H.L., Hanna, A.K., Marliss, E.B., Vranic, M., & Zinman, B. (1980). Metabolic response to moderate exercise in obese man during prolonged fasting. *American Journal of Physiology, 238*(4), E322-E329.

Minuk, H.L., Vranic, M., Marliss, E.B., Hanna, A.K., Albisser, A.M., & Zinman, B. (1981). Glucoregulatory and metabolic response to exercise in obese non-insulin-dependent diabetes. *American Journal of Physiology, 240*(5), E458-E464.

Mustonen, J.N., Uusitupa, M.I., Tahvanainen, K., Talwar, S., Laakso, M., Lansimies, E., Kuikka, J.T., & Pyorala, K. (1988). Impaired left ventricular systolic function during exercise in middle-aged insulin-dependent and non-insulin-dependent diabetic subjects without clinically evident cardiovascular disease. *American Journal of Cardiology, 1:62*(17), 1273-1279.

Naka, M., Hiramatsu, K., Aizawa, T., Momose, A., Yoshizawa, K., Shigematsu, S., Ishihara, F., Niwa, A., & Yamada, T. (1992). Silent myocardial ischemia in patients with non-insulin-dependent diabetes mellitus as judged by treadmill exercise testing and coronary angiography. *American Heart Journal*, **123**(1), 46-53.

Nesher, R., Karl, I.E., & Kipnis, K.M. (1985). Dissociation of the effects of insulin and contraction on glucose transport in rat epitrochlearis muscle. *American Journal of Physiology*, **249**, C226-C232.

Obermaier-Kusser, B., White, M.F., Pongratz, D.E., Su, Z., Ermel, B., Muhlbacher, C., & Harin, H.U. (1989). A defective intramolecular autoactivation cascade may cause the reduced kinase activity of the skeletal muscle insulin receptor from patients with non-insulin-dependent diabetes mellitus. *Journal of Biological Chemistry*, **264**, 9497-9504.

Paternostro-Bayles, M., Wing, R.R., & Robertson, R.J. (1989). Effect of lifestyle activity of varying duration on glycemic control in Type II diabetic women. *Diabetes Care*, **12**, 34-37.

Pedersen, O., Bak, J.S., Andersen, P.H., Lund, S., Moller, D.E., Flier, J.S., & Kahn, B.B. (1990). Evidence against altered expression of GLUT 1 or GLUT 4 in skeletal muscle of patients with obesity or NIDDM. *Diabetes*, **39**, 865-870.

Price, T.B., Rothman, D.L., Avison, M.J., Buonamico, P., & Shulman, R.G. (1991). 13CNMR measurements of muscle glycogen during low-intensity exercise. *Journal of Applied Physiology*, **70**(4), 1836-1844.

Richter, E.A., Turcotte, L., Hespel, P., & Kiens, B. (1992). Metabolic responses to exercise: Effects of endurance training and implications for diabetes. *Diabetes Care*, **15**(Suppl. 4), 1767-1776.

Rodnick, K.J., Piper, R.C., Slot, J.W., & James, D.E. (1992). Interaction of insulin and exercise on glucose transport in muscle. *Diabetes Care*, **15**(Suppl. 4), 1679-1689.

Rogers, M.A., Yamamoto, C., King, D., Hagberg, J.M., Ehsani, A.A., & Holloszy, J.O. (1988). Improvement in glucose tolerance after 1 week of exercise in patients with mild NIDDM. *Diabetes Care*, **11**(8), 613-618.

Romanelli, G., Giustina, A., Agabiti-Rosei, E., Bossoni, S., Girelli, A., Muiesan, M.L., Muiesan, G., & Giustina, G. (1989). Short-term use of Captopril and Nifedipine on microalbuminuria induced by exercise in hypertensive diabetic patients. *Journal of Hypertension Supplement*, **7**(6), S312-S313.

Sacca, L., Morrone, G., Cicala, M., Corso, G., & Ungaro, B. (1980). Influence of epinephrine, norepinephrine and isoproterenol on glucose homeostasis in normal man. *Journal of Clinical Endocrinology and Metabolism*, **50**, 680-684.

Sahlin, K. (1990). Muscle glucose metabolism during exercise. *Annals of Medicine*, **22**(3), 85-89.

Schneider, S.H., Khachadurian, A.K., Amorosa, L.F., Gavras, H., Fineberg, S.E., & Ruderman, N.B. (1987). Abnormal glucoregulation during exercise in Type II (non-insulin-dependent) diabetes. *Metabolism*, **36**(12), 1161-1166.

Schneider, S.H., Kim, H.C., Khachadurian, A.K., & Ruderman, N.B. (1988). Effects of exercise and physical training. *Metabolism*, **37**(10), 924-929.

Sternlicht, E., Barnard, R.J., & Grimditch, G.K. (1989). Exercise and insulin stimulate skeletal muscle glucose transport through different mechanisms. *American Journal of Physiology*, **256**, E227-E230.

Takahashi, N., Iwasaka, T., Sugiura, T., Hasegawa, T., Tarumi, N., & Inada, M. (1991). Diastolic time in diabetes. Impairment of diastolic time during dynamic exercise in Type 2 diabetes with retinopathy. *Chest*, **100**(3), 748-753.

Takahashi, N., Iwasaka, T., Sugiura, T., Hasegawa, T., Tarumi, N., Matsutani, M., Onoyama, H., & Inada, M. (1991). Left ventricular dysfunction during dynamic exercise in noninsulin-dependent diabetic patients with retinopathy. *Cardiology*, **78**(1), 23-30.

Torgan, C.E., Brozinick, J.T., Jr., Willems, M.E., & Ivy, J.L. (1990). Substrate utilization during acute exercise in obese Zucker rats. *Journal of Applied Physiology*, **69**(6), 1987-1991.

Treadway, J.L., James, D.E., Burcel, E., & Ruderman, N.B. (1989). Effect of exercise on insulin receptor binding and kinase activity in skeletal muscle. *American Journal of Physiology*, **256**, E138-E144.

Vranic, M., & Berger, M. (1979). Exercise and diabetes mellitus. *Diabetes*, **28**, 147-163.

Wahren, J., Felig, P., Ahlborg, G., & Jorfeldt, L. (1971). Glucose metabolism during leg exercise in man. *Journal of Clinical Investigation*, **50**, 2715-2725.

Wallberg-Henriksson, H. (1987). Glucose transport into skeletal muscle. Influence of contractile activity, insulin, catecholamines and diabetes mellitus. *Acta Physiologica Scandinavica*, **131**(Suppl.), 1-80.

Wallberg-Henriksson, H. (1992). Interaction of exercise and insulin in Type II diabetes mellitus. *Diabetes Care*, **15**(4), 1777-1782.

Wallberg-Henriksson, H., & Holloszy, J.O. (1985). Activation of glucose transport in diabetic muscle: Responses to contraction and insulin. *American Journal of Physiology*, **249**, C233-C237.

Wasserman, D.H., Geer, R.J., Rice, D.E., Bracy, D., Flakoll, P.J., Brown, L.L., Hill, J.O., & Abumrad, N.N. (1991). Interaction of exercise and insulin action in humans. *American Journal of Physiology*, **260**(1 Pt. 1), E37-E45.

Wasserman, D.H., Lacy, D.B., Goldstein, R.E., Williams, P.E., & Cherrington, A.D. (1989). Exercise-induced fall in insulin and increase in fat metabolism during prolonged muscular work. *Diabetes*, **38**(4), 484-490.

Wasserman, D.H., Lickley, H.L., & Vranic, M. (1985). Important role of glucagon during exercise in diabetic dogs. *Journal of Applied Physiology*, **59**(4), 1272-1281.

Wasserman, D.H., Spalding, J.A., Bracy, D., Lacy, D.B., & Cherrington, A.D. (1989). Exercise-induced rise in glucagon and ketogenesis during prolonged muscular work. *Diabetes,* **38**(6), 799-807.

Wasserman, D.H., Spalding, J.A., Lacy, D.B., Colburn, C.A., Goldstein, R.E., & Cherrington, A.D. (1989). Glucagon is a primary controller of hepatic glycogenolysis and gluconeogenesis during muscular work. *American Journal of Physiology,* **257**(1 Pt. 1), E108-E117.

Wasserman, D.H., Williams, P.E., Lacy, D.B., Goldstein, R.E., & Cherrington, A.D. (1989). Exercise-induced fall in insulin and hepatic carbohydrate metabolism during muscular work. *American Journal of Physiology,* **256**(4 Pt. 1), E500-E509.

Wolfe, R.R., Goodenough, R.D., Wolfe, M.H., Royle, G.T., & Nadel, E.R. (1982). Isotopic analysis of leucine and urea metabolism in exercising humans. *Journal of Applied Physiology,* **52**(2), 458-466.

Yale, J.F., Leiter, L.A., & Marliss, E.B. (1989). Metabolic responses to intense exercise in lean and obese subjects. *Journal of Clinical Endocrinology and Metabolism,* **68**(2), 438-445.

Chapter 5

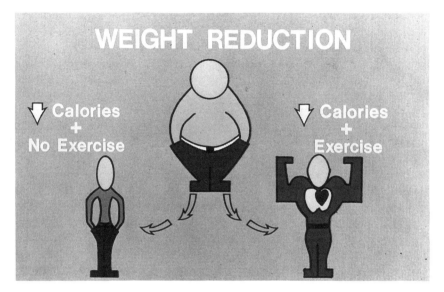

Physical Training in the Management of Type II Diabetes

Physical training, or habitual muscle contractile activity, involves the regular performance of a specific exercise over a period of weeks during which the body adapts to the stresses induced. This adaptation process involves numerous physiological responses, including cardiovascular, metabolic, neural, and hormonal, to name a few. In this chapter, the significant physiological adaptations to physical training that have been found to occur in people with Type II diabetes will be described and discussed.

Physical Training in People Without Diabetes

Exercise training is a state that represents an accumulation of acute exercise bouts performed over a period of time where physiological adaptations are manifested. Endurance training in people without diabetes has been shown to increase insulin sensitivity. The potential benefits of exercise training in insulin-resistant states may result from the additive responses of acute exercise, especially if it is intense enough to produce marked glycogen depletion in skeletal muscle. Exercise training increases glucose transport and metabolism (Bonen, Clune, & Tan, 1986; Tan & Bonen, 1987; Wallberg-Henrikksson, 1986), but this effect may be lost within 2 days after training is stopped (Burstein et al., 1985; Heath et al., 1983). Exercise training may enhance insulin-mediated glucose uptake and may improve oral glucose tolerance, even in the presence of lower insulin concentration in response to an oral glucose challenge. However, the effects of exercise in improving glucose tolerance and insulin resistance may be the short-term effects of the last bout of exercise. In nondiabetic athletes, glucose tolerance deteriorated within 10 days of cessation of exercise (Heath et al.), and insulin-mediated glucose uptake disappeared within 60 hr of the last bout of exercise (Burstein et al., 1985). These findings suggest that the effects of exercise training are the result of repeated acute effects of exercise. But other studies (Davis et al., 1986; Mikines, Sonne, Farrell, Tronier, & Galbo, 1988; Wallberg-Henrikkson, 1986; Young, Enslin, & Kuca, 1989) suggest that trained muscle with adequate insulin present displays an increased capacity to metabolize glucose rather than reflecting the residual effects of the last bout of acute exercise. Recent work by Bonen, Tan, Megeney, and McDermott (1992) examined whether enhanced glucose metabolism in muscle of trained animals reflected training adaptations or residual effects of acute exercise. These investigators reported that an acute bout of exercise increased glycogenesis, whereas training increased glycolysis. They concluded that exercise training does cause adaptations in glucose metabolism and that these adaptations differ from changes resulting from the last bout of acute exercise.

    In the physically trained state, hepatic tissue gives priority to glucose synthesis and storage in muscles during postexercise recovery (Rodnick, Haskell, Swislocki, Foley, & Reaven, 1987; Yki-Jarvinen & Koivisto, 1983). Glucose tolerance is improved even in the presence of reduced insulin levels in nondiabetic individuals (Mikines et al., 1988; Rodnick et al., 1987). Muscle, liver, and adipose tissue show enhanced insulin sensitivity in trained distance runners as compared with nontrained runners (Rodnick et al.). Hepatic glucose production rates during euglycemic hyperinsulinemic tests with blood infusion levels at either 10 $\mu u/ml$ or 50 $\mu u/ml$ have been shown to be reduced in people who are physically trained (Rodnick et al.). Insulin resistance, as measured by mean glucose concentrations during an insulin sensitivity test (euglycemic hyperinsulinemic clamp technique), has been reported to decrease with exercise training in subjects with hypertriglyceridemia only from 140 ± 11.7 to 103 ± 11.3 mg/dl ($p < 0.01$), indicating improved insulin-mediated glucose uptake (Lampman et al., 1985).

If improvements in glucose tolerance and insulin resistance are to be maintained, exercise training must be performed regularly. Exercise training, used as a therapeutic modality alone or in combination with diet, insulin, or oral hypoglycemic agents, may have major effects on circulating concentrations of glucose, insulin, lipids, and lipoproteins. This chapter focuses on reviewing exercise training for achieving euglycemia, enhancing insulin sensitivity, improving oral glucose tolerance, and improving plasma lipids.

Physical Training in Type II Diabetes

Abnormalities in glucose tolerance, increased plasma insulin levels, and resistance to insulin action due to receptor or postreceptor defects (or both) are major metabolic disorders that characterize patients with NIDDM. The causes of cellular insulin resistance can be due to many factors, including

- reduced number or altered structure or function of the insulin receptor (Taylor et al., 1990),
- reduced glucose transporter number and activity (Kahn, Charron, Lodish, Cushman, & Flier, 1989), and
- reduced intracellular enzyme activity (Mandarino, Consoli, Thorne, & Kelley, 1988).

Additional research is needed to understand the effects of muscular contractions and exercise training in improving cellular insulin sensitivity and insulin-mediated glucose uptake in respect to these abnormalities. Furthermore, these abnormalities often are associated with elevated levels of very low-density lipoprotein triglyceride (VLDL-TG) and low-density lipoprotein cholesterol (LDL-Chol) and with reduced high-density lipoprotein cholesterol (HDL-Chol) blood concentrations. Usually, patients with NIDDM are overweight (Holbrook, Barrett-Connor, & Wingard, 1989).

The recommendation to use exercise training therapeutically to lower glucose and lipid levels in people with Type II diabetes (National Institutes of Health, 1987) stems from the pronounced effects of acute exercise on the metabolism of glucose, insulin, and lipids (Ahlborg, Felig, Hagenfeldt, Hendler, & Wahren, 1974; Wahren, Felig, Ahlborg, & Horfeldt, 1971). Importantly, exercise training has been shown to improve insulin sensitivity in those with Type II diabetes (Holloszy, Schultz, Kusnierkiewicz, Hagberg, & Ehsani, 1986; Reitman, Vasquez, Klimes, & Hagulesparan, 1984; Trovati et al., 1984), probably as a result of enhanced insulin action in skeletal muscle (James, Kraegen, & Chisholm, 1985; Mondon, Dolkas, & Reaven, 1980). Furthermore, inactivity rapidly reverses the effects of training on insulin metabolism (Burstein et al., 1985), and the prevalence of

Type II diabetes is more than twice as high in sedentary men than in a matched group of active men (Taylor, Ram, Zimmet, Raper, & Ringrose, 1984).

The possible therapeutic benefits of exercise training for people with NIDDM include the following:

- Reduced blood glucose and insulin levels
- Improved oral glucose tolerance
- Improved insulin secretion response to oral glucose stimulus
- Improved peripheral and hepatic insulin sensitivity
- Improved blood lipid and lipoprotein concentrations
- Decreased hypertension
- Reduced risk for advanced cardiovascular disease
- Increased physical fitness level
- Increased caloric expenditure contributing to weight reduction/ maintenance
- Enhanced quality of life
- Healthier lifestyle
- Increased sense of well-being

Glucose Control, Basal Glucose Levels, Oral and IV Glucose Tolerance

Improvements in diabetic control as assessed by fasting plasma glucose levels were demonstrated in 5 NIDDM patients following a 6-week exercise training program that resulted in a 15% increase in $\dot{V}O_2$max (Trovati et al., 1984). Reitman et al. (1984) also reported improvement of glucose homeostasis in individuals with NIDDM who train 5 to 6 times per week for 6 to 10 weeks. Therapeutic strategies involving a combination of both exercise and weight reduction also improved fasting plasma glucose concentrations (Bogardus et al., 1984; Wing et al., 1988). Changes in basal glucose levels may not be transient because exercise training has been shown to reduce HbA_{1c} levels in people with Type II diabetes (Schneider, Amorosa, Khachadurian, & Ruderman, 1984; Rönnemaa, Mattilla, Lehtonen, & Kallio, 1986; Ruderman, Ganda, & Johansen, 1979; Trovati et al., 1984). Improved glycemic control may be associated with the cumulative effect of frequent high-intensity acute exercise that results in lowering blood glucose levels (Koivisto, Yki-Jarvinen, & DeFronzo, 1986; Schneider et al., 1984), and improvements may be seen within a week of beginning intense exercise (Rogers et al., 1988). Skeletal muscle is the primary tissue responsible for increased glucose disposal during the postexercise period as a result of enhanced glucose transport and augmented glycogen synthesis, resulting in reduced plasma glucose levels. Minuk et al. (1981) reported a fall in glucose during a 45-min exercise session at 60% $\dot{V}O_2$max in patients with NIDDM. The fall occurred because the hepatic glucose production was reduced while peripheral glucose utilization increased normally as a result of abnormally elevated insulin secretion. In the study by Schneider et al. (1984) a 12% reduction in HbA_{1c} was reported for a group of middle-aged patients with Type II diabetes in a hospital-based exercise training program for 6 weeks. Glucose tolerance remained improved after the last bout of exercise in these patients at 12 and 17 hr, but not 3 days later. Rather than changes in HbA_{1c} being associated with improvements in $\dot{V}O_2max$, they related to the cumulative effect of the individual exercise bouts. This may be why other researchers have reported no change in overall oral and intravenous glucose tolerance in people with Type II diabetes, even though improvements in $\dot{V}O_2max$ followed exercise training (Krotkiewski et al., 1985; Schneider et al., 1984). Rönnemaa et al. (1986) reported that an exercise training program for patients with mild to moderate NIDDM lowered the 2-hr plasma glucose level and markedly increased plasma insulin and C-peptide responses during an oral glucose challenge.

Exercise training for patients with NIDDM has not always improved glucose tolerance and plasma insulin levels (Ruderman et al., 1979; Saltin et al., 1979; Schneider et al., 1984; Trovati et al., 1984). Huh et al. (1986) have reported that exercise training over a period of 14 weeks to 34 weeks was ineffective in improving fasting plasma glucose levels or oral glucose tolerance in middle-aged, moderately obese subjects with NIDDM. These authors found that exercise training without weight loss was ineffective in reducing fasting glucose, insulin, and lipid levels and for improving oral glucose tolerance in subjects with NIDDM. To be most effective, exercise training may need to be high intensity and the individual may need a calorie-restricted diet. Lampman and Schteingart (1991) have demonstrated marked improvements in glucose metabolism in obese subjects undergoing a program of both exercise and hypocaloric intake. These improvements were greater than those found in similar subjects receiving diet therapy alone. This work supports the premise that the addition of exercise to a hypocaloric diet can greatly enhance the beneficial effect of diet on glucose metabolism in insulin-resistant states in overweight people.

Improved blood glucose levels through physical training alone or in combination with diet have been demonstrated in young and middle-aged individuals with Type II diabetes (Bogardus et al., 1984; Krotkiewski et al., 1985; Reitman et al., 1984; Ruderman et al., 1979). Vanninen, Uusitupa, Siitonen, Laitinen, & Länsimies (1992) recently reported that middle-aged obese Type II patients displayed an inverse relationship between aerobic capacity and HbA_{1c} levels after a 12-month hypocaloric diet and exercise program. Both body weight and HbA_{1c} levels decreased by 23%. These studies suggest that exercise training in combination with weight loss might be necessary to effectively lower glucose levels and help maintain long-term glycemic control in obese patients with NIDDM (Lampman et al., 1987; Skarfors, Wegener, Lithel, & Selinus, 1987).

Holloszy et al. (1986) demonstrated that exercise is effective in normalizing oral glucose tolerance only in those patients who are still able to secrete insulin and in those patients who display peripheral insulin resistance. To improve glycemic control in this study, a high level of training—running 25 to 35 km per week at a speed that elicits at least 70% to 80% of $\dot{V}O_2$max—was necessary. Animal studies involving severely diabetic rats have demonstrated that physical training may not improve intravenous glucose tolerance when the disease is in advanced stages (Vallerand, Lupien, Deshaies, & Bukowieki, 1986).

Improved glycemic control through exercise training that improves $\dot{V}O_2$max is best accomplished in individuals with mild Type II diabetes who are hyperinsulinemic but have fasting glucose levels less than 200 mg/dl (Rogers et al., 1988; Rönnemaa et al., 1986; Schneider et al., 1984; Trovati et al., 1984). The major implication of this finding is that these patients secrete more insulin than people with more severe hyperglycemia and that hyperinsulinemia is reduced with exercise training (Holloszy et al., 1986; Rogers et al., 1988).

Insulin Secretion

Because of the heterogeneity of insulin-resistant states, responses to exercise training may differ among individuals. Whether improvements in insulin sensitivity occur with exercise may depend on the initial basal-insulin levels and whether improved glucose levels are associated with increased insulin secretion (DeFronzo, 1988; Krotkiewski et al., 1985; Rönnemaa et al., 1986; Unger & Grundy, 1985). Krotkiewski et al. demonstrated a reduced rate of insulin secretion in individuals with initially high levels of insulin secretion, as assessed by elevated levels of C-peptide, and an improvement in peripheral insulin sensitivity in response to 3 months of physical training without weight loss. These subjects showed no concomitant improvement in glucose tolerance. In comparison, NIDDM individuals displaying insulin resistance, but initially low insulin secretion rates, increased the rate of insulin secretion with training (Krotkiewski et al., 1985). An increased hepatic breakdown of insulin was suspected because peripheral insulin concentrations were unchanged. Glucose tolerance did improve in this latter group of patients due to an increase in peripheral insulin sensitivity.

Reitman et al. (1984) studied 6 obese patients with NIDDM for glucose tolerance, insulin secretory capacity, and insulin glucose disposal following 6 to 10 weeks of intensive aerobic exercise training. In this study, subjects maintained body weight. Their fasting plasma glucose declined, on average, 33 mg/dl, and oral glucose tolerance improved in 5 of the 6 subjects. Improvements in plasma glucose levels were highly correlated to the degrees of hyperglycemia before training and closely correlated with observed improvements in the early (30-min) plasma insulin secretion in response to an oral glucose challenge. Improvements in peripheral insulin resistance, as assessed by the euglycemic clamp technique, did not occur. Trovati et al. (1984) investigated the influence of physical training on blood glucose control, glucose tolerance, insulin secretion, and insulin action in five patients with NIDDM. This 6-week program of daily exercise for 1 hr at 50% to 60% maximum oxygen uptake improved blood glucose levels, oral glucose tolerance, and insulin action. Results of this study suggest that intense physical training, even though short term, can improve metabolic abnormalities associated with NIDDM.

Peripheral and Hepatic Insulin Sensitivity

Exercise training may improve insulin-stimulated glucose disposal rate in patients with NIDDM (Krotkiewski et al., 1985; Trovati et al., 1984). Peripheral insulin sensitivity, as measured by glucose disposal during the hyperinsulinemic euglycemic clamp test, has been reported to improve with exercise training in some studies (Koivisto & DeFronzo, 1984; Krotkiewski et al., Trovati et al., Bogardus et al., 1984). Improved insulin-stimulated glucose uptake has not been a universal finding because exercise training alone has not always been shown to improve skeletal muscle insulin sensitivity in insulin-resistant states (Crettaz, Horton, Warzala, Horton, & Jeanrenaud, 1983; Ivy, Sherman, Cutler, & Katz, 1986; Lampman et al., 1987).

If an insulin-resistant state exists, intense exercise training, exercise training in combination with a high-carbohydrate diet (Vallerand, Lupien, & Bukowlecki, 1986) or exercise training plus a diet high in complex carbohydrates (Ivy, et al., 1986), may be necessary to improve skeletal muscle insulin sensitivity. Evidence from animal studies also suggests that for exercise to favorably affect metabolic control, a minimal concentration of circulating insulin is required (Schneider et al., 1984).

Holloszy et al. (1986) studied the effects of vigorous exercise training on glucose tolerance and insulin resistance in subjects with mild NIDDM and in those with impaired glucose tolerance. Improved insulin sensitivity and glucose tolerance occurred only in individuals who still had adequate capacity to secrete insulin and in those individuals who displayed insulin resistance. These results also showed that it is necessary to perform at least 25 to 35 km of running per week to normalize glucose tolerance. This suggests that improvements in insulin sensitivity by people with diabetes undergoing exercise training may depend on the severity of the initial metabolic state and whether the patient undergoing exercise training can markedly increase maximum oxygen consumption. Lampman et al. (1987) have shown that exercise training increased oxygen consumption in patients with Type II diabetes from 29.7 ± 1.0 ml/kg/min to 34.2 ± 1.4 ml/kg/min ($p < 0.01$) without improvements noted in glucose tolerance or in vivo insulin sensitivity. It is important to note that the initial oxygen consumption values found among subjects in this study were approximately 4.5 ml/kg/min lower than those found in euglycemic, hypertriglyceridemic subjects of a similar age (Lampman et al., 1985). Although the abnormal glucose response to oral glucose did not change with training, insulin concentrations were significantly lower at 90 and 120 min during the final oral glucose tolerance test, suggesting that exercise may alter the late insulin release phase. In vivo insulin sensitivity, measured by the euglycemic hyperinsulinemic clamp technique, also did not change in these glucose intolerant, nonobese, hypertriglyceridemic subjects following exercise training. The glucose utilization rate was 3.1 ± 0.8 mg/kg/min at baseline and 2.9 ± 1.2 mg/kg/min after the physical training program. These results suggest that a V̇O₂max threshold may exist that must be achieved to help ameliorate abnormalities in glucose and insulin metabolism.

Segal et al. (1991) studied the effects of exercise training on insulin sensitivity and glucose metabolism in lean, obese, and diabetic men. Subjects performed a cycle ergometry exercise program 4 hr per week at approximately 70% of maximum oxygen uptake for 12 weeks. An attempt was made to maintain body weight by replacing the energy expended in each training session. Euglycemic hyperinsulinemic clamps were performed at a plasma glucose level of 90 mg/dl. Indirect calorimetry measured substrate utilization. Residual hepatic glucose output was calculated to correct for total insulin-stimulated glucose disposal. Cardiovascular fitness increased by 27% in all groups. Body weight, fat, and fat free mass did not change with exercise training. Both before and after training, the metabolic clearance rate of glucose was lower for the obese men as compared to the lean men, and lower for the diabetic men than the obese. Insulin sensitivity was not improved by training in any group. However, hepatic glucose production was reduced by 22% in the diabetic men. The authors conclude that when studying the intervening effects of exercise training, the last bout of exercise, changes in body composition, or both must be considered. Not all investigators agree that exercise training alters hepatic glucose production and suggest that this tissue does not improve its insulin sensitivity (Horton, 1988).

Subjects with Type II diabetes mellitus may need to achieve a fitness threshold with improved cardiovascular variables to normalize glucose tolerance. Bjorntorp & Krotkiewski (1985) reported that physical training produced limited improvements in glucose tolerance in subjects with NIDDM. They hypothesize that there may not be a normal compensatory increase in glucose release from hepatic sources during exercise in these patients, possibly due to higher plasma insulin concentrations that do not decrease during exercise as they do in healthy individuals (Minuk et al., 1981). If reduced hepatic release of glucose were to occur, it could cause hypoglycemia that in turn would influence the ability to exercise at a sufficient intensity and duration to lead to a physically trained state. The authors reported that subjects with low insulin secretion improved most in glucose tolerance. They suggested that enhanced insulin secretion resulting from physical training may have influenced hepatic insulin sensitivity, and that increased muscle sensitivity to insulin, as well as peripheral insulin resistance, improved. Table 5.1 shows an overview of reports measuring the effects of exercise training on peripheral insulin sensitivity.

Adipose Tissue

Animal studies have demonstrated increases in glucose metabolism in adipose tissue in response to exercise training (James et al., 1985; Wardzala, Crettaz, Horton, Jeanrenaud, & Horton, 1982) by

- increased insulin-stimulated glucose uptake;
- enhanced transport, intracellular metabolism, and incorporation into fatty acids; and
- increased sensitivity of lipolysis to epinephrine.

These findings may in part be due to an increased number of glucose transporters in plasma membrane fractions and a decrease in the low-density microsomes (Vinten, Norgaad-Peterson, Slonne, & Galbo, 1985), reduced adipocyte cell size (Craig, Garthwaite, & Holloszy, 1987), and an improvement in postreceptor events rather than an improvement in insulin binding (Wardzala et al., 1982).

Skeletal Muscle

Skeletal muscle tissue adaptations to exercise training in Type II diabetes are an important consideration because this tissue is thought to play a major role in peripheral insulin resistance characteristic of this disease. Muscle capillary density and fiber type have been suggested as determinants of in vivo insulin resistance (Lillioja et al., 1987). Evidence from animal studies suggests that exercise training can increase capillary density, which may be the mechanism for improved muscle insulin sensitivity (James, Burleigh, Storlien, Bennett, & Kraegen, 1986). Muscle capillary density has been shown to increase with physical training in healthy individuals (Andersen & Henriksson, 1977). Conflicting results regarding whether patients with NIDDM increase muscle capillary density in response to physical training have been reported (Allenberg, Johansen, & Salton, 1988; Lithell et al., 1985). These discrepancies may be due to vascular lesions associated with diabetes, to differences in training protocols, or both (Allenberg et al.; Lithell et al.) Improvements in VO_2max and skeletal muscle oxidative enzyme activity in people with Type II diabetes have occurred with exercise training (Allenberg et al.; Krotkiewski et al., 1985; Lithell et al.) just as they have in healthy people (Henriksson & Reitman, 1977). (See Table 5.2.)

Rather than being an adaptive change occuring with physical training, altered glucose uptake by muscle may reflect an acute response to exercise.

Table 5.1 Effects of Exercise Training on Insulin Sensitivity in Type II Diabetes

Author	Patients	Exercise program	Diet	Changes in $\dot{V}O_2$max	Insulin sensitivity
Lampman et al., 1985	Nondiabetic ($N = 10$), non-obese (82.3 ± 4.3 kg), hypertriglyceridemic, middle-aged men (44.5 ± 0.8 yr)	Moderate to strenuous, 85% HR_{max}, 30-40 min, 3 × week, 9 weeks	Isocaloric	33.5 ± 1.9 to 39.3 ± 1.9 ml · kg (17% improvement)	Improved
Soman et al., 1979	Nondiabetic ($N = 6$), non-obese (74.1 ± 4.3 kg), healthy, young men (25 ± 2 yr)	Moderate to strenuous, 70% $\dot{V}O_2$max, 60 min, 4 × week, 6 weeks	Isocaloric	42.6 ± 0.9 to 50.8 ± 2.3 ml · kg · min (19% improvement)	Improved
Schteingart et al., 1985	Nondiabetic ($N = 20$) and NIDDM ($N = 15$), severely obese (132 ± 7.1 kg), young and middle-aged (20-60 yr) men ($N = 10$) and women ($N = 25$)	Moderate, 75% HR_{max}, 45 min, 3 × week, 24 weeks	Hypocaloric (600 kcal · d)		
	Nondiabetic ($N = 9$)			16.9 ± 1.7 to 25.0 ± 2.1 ml · kg · min (49% improvement)	Improved
	NIDDM ($N = 7$)			15.1 ± 0.89 to 20.0 ± 2.1 ml · kg · min (36% improvement)	Improved

Study	Subjects	Exercise program	Diet	$\dot{V}O_2$max	Insulin sensitivity
Lampman et al., 1987	Glucose intolerant (N = 14) and NIDDM (N = 5), nonobese (81.0 ± 3.9 kg), hypertriglyceridemic, middle-aged men (48.9 ± 0.5 yr)	Moderate to strenuous, 85% HR_{max}, 30-40 min, 3 × week, 9 weeks	Isocaloric	29.7 ± 1.0 to 34.2 ± 1.4 ml · kg · min (15% improvement)	No change
Trovati et al., 1984	NIDDM (N = 5), nonobese (82 ± 6 kg), middle-aged men (54 ± 4 yr)	Strenuous, 50%-60% $\dot{V}O_2$max, 60 min daily, 6 weeks	Isocaloric (400 kcal extra per day)	2018 ± 98 to 2348 ± 107 ml · min (24.6 to 28.6 ml · kg · min)* (15% improvement)	Improved
Reitman et al., 1984	NIDDM (N = 6), obese (106.0 ± 4.9 kg), American Indian, young (26.3 ± 3.2 yr) men (N = 3) and women (N = 3)	Strenuous, 60%-90%, $\dot{V}O_2$max, 20-40 min, 5-6 × week, 6-10 weeks	Isocaloric: 45% CHO, 35% fat, 20% protein	40.0 ± 2.0 to 46.5 ± 1.5 ml · kg FFM · min (26.6 ± 1.2 to 31.0 ± 1.5 ml · kg · min) (17% improvement)	No change
Bogardus et al. (1984)	NIDDM and glucose intolerant (N = 10), obese (98.2 ± 6.6 kg), middle-aged (44 ± 11 yr) men (N = 2) and women (N = 8)	Moderate, 75% HR_{max}, 20-30 min, 3 × week, 1-12 weeks	Hypocaloric (450 kcal · m^{-2}): 60% CHO, 15% fat, 25% protein	37.0 ± 0.92 to 41.8 ± 0.9 ml · kg FFM^{-1} · min^{-1}* (23.5 to 28.7 ml · kg^{-1} · min^{-1})* (13% improvement)	Improved

FFM = fat-free mass

*Calculated from data published in paper.

From "Effects of Exercise Training on Glucose Control, Lipid Metabolism, and Insulin Sensitivity in Hypertriglyceridemia and Non-Insulin-Dependent Diabetes Mellitus" by R.M. Lampman and D.E. Schteingart, 1991, *Medicine and Science in Sports and Exercise*, **23**(6), pp. 703-712. Copyright 1991 by Williams and Wilkins, Inc. Reprinted by permission.

Table 5.2   Changes in Skeletal Muscle in Response to Physical Training in Insulin-Resistant States

Measure	Change
Capillary density	Increase/decrease
Oxidative enzymes	
Citrate synthase	Increase
Succinate dehydrogenase	Increase
3-Hydroxyacyl-CoA	Increase
Lactate dehydrogenase	None
Intramuscular glycogen	Increase
Glucose uptake	Increase
Glycogen synthesis	Increase

Animal studies suggest that muscle glucose uptake reflects the residual effects of the last exercise session rather than an adaptation in skeletal muscle insulin sensitivity to training (Ivy, Young, McLane, Fell, & Holloszy, 1983). Studies in healthy individuals show that acute exercise increases insulin binding to monocytes due to increased receptor affinity (Michel, Vocke, Flehn, Weicker, Schwarz, & Bieger, 1984), but little is known about whether muscle cells respond in a similar manner. Even if skeletal muscle adaptations to physical training occur in people with Type II diabetes, no effect on glucose homeostasis or lipaemia may occur (Allenberg et al., 1988). Lactate dehydrogenase activity, a marker of glycolytic metabolism, does not change in people with Type II diabetes or normal controls in response to exercise training (Allenberg et al., 1988).

Exercise training in obese Zucker rats has been shown to result in favorable skeletal morphological and biochemical changes such as an increase in oxidative enzymes and an increase in capillary density (Torgan, Brozinick, Kastello, & Ivy, 1989). In this animal model, exercise training improves the glucose transport process and is fiber type specific (Ivy, Brozinick, Torgan, & Kastello, 1989). The intensity of exercise during training may be an important factor for improved insulin-stimulated glucose transport in skeletal muscle. Cortez, Torgan, Brozinick, and Ivy (1991) found that high-intensity training in insulin-resistant obese Zucker rats resulted in a marked enhancement of 3-0-methyl-D-glucose of fast-twitch white muscle fibers. Obese Zucker rats demonstrated reduced glucose transport in slow-twitch, oxidative fibers of soleus muscle; in fast-twitch, oxidative, glycolytic fibers of red quadriceps; and in mixed fibers of gastrocnemius muscle when compared with lean rats (Sherman, Katz, Cutler, Withers, & Ivy, 1988). Exercise training may be beneficial in altering skeletal muscle glucose uptake because maximal skeletal muscle glucose uptake in obese Zucker rats is not resistant to stimulation by contractile activity, despite resistance to the glucose uptake stimulation by insulin (Brozinick, Etgen, Yaspelkis, & Ivy, 1992).

Muscle strips from Type II diabetic subjects, studied in vitro, show a marked reduction in glucose transport in response to a high concentration of insulin as compared with tissue from nondiabetic individuals (Andréasson, Galuska, Thörne, Sonnenfield, & Wallberg-Henriksson, 1991). This finding suggests insulin postreceptor defects in those with NIDDM, perhaps multiple in nature, that may depend on the severity of diabetes, the degree of obesity, or both (Arner, Pollare, Lithell, & Livingston, 1987; Caro, Dohm, Pories, & Sinha, 1989; Caro et al., 1987; Obermaier-Kusser, White, Pongratz, Su, & Ermel, 1989; Pedersen et al., 1990).

Wallberg-Henriksson (1986) investigated the ability of muscle to act as a regulator of glucose transport through repeated muscle contractions using an isolated rat epitrochlearis muscle preparation. Baseline measures of glucose transport in muscles from rats with streptozocin-induced diabetes were 52% lower than normal controls. Following a 3-day period of swimming, muscles from diabetic rats displayed normal contraction-induced and insulin-stimulated glucose transport capacity. These results demonstrate that repeated contractile activity can improve insulin sensitivity. A major defect in the impairment of insulin to affect normal glucose disposal in muscle has been attributed to the reduction of the major insulin-sensitive glucose transporter, Glut 4 (Douen, Ramlal, Cartee, & Klip, 1990; Douen, Ramlal, Rastogi, et al., 1990). Others have not demonstrated that this glucose transporter has an abnormal expression in NIDDM patients (Pedersen et al., 1990). Conditions or possible mechanisms for a decrease in glucose transport in skeletal muscle of individuals with Type II diabetes are

Obese

- decreased insulin binding,
- decreased insulin receptor number,
- decreased insulin receptor tyrosine kinase activity, and
- decreased glucose transporter protein;

Nonobese

- no alteration in glucose transporters.

Maximal Oxygen Consumption

Lampman et al. (1987) have reported lower peak $\dot{V}O_2$max levels in patients with NIDDM as compared with matched controls before training. Others have also noted lower than normal $\dot{V}O_2$max levels in individuals with Type II diabetes (Schneider et al., 1984). No change was found in $\dot{V}O_2$max after a year of unsupervised home exercise in Type II subjects (Vanninen et al., 1992). Others have reported that exercise training has improved functional capacity as measured by improvements in $\dot{V}O_2$max in people with Type II diabetes (Lampman et al., 1987; Ruderman et al., 1979; Schneider et al., 1984; Verity & Ismail, 1989). Allenberg et al. (1988) found a 10% increase in $\dot{V}O_2$max in those with Type II diabetes after physical training. Rönnemaa et al. (1986) reported that NIDDM patients with the poorest metabolic control prior to exercise training failed to improve their physical fitness levels or their metabolic control after training. This lack of improved physical fitness and metabolic control may stem from the inability of these patients to achieve exercise intensity high enough to exert beneficial effects. Hence, whereas physical training may improve $\dot{V}O_2$max in people with NIDDM, $\dot{V}O_2$max threshold may need to be achieved to accomplish optimal glycemic control (Lampman et al., 1987). Improved fitness levels, similar to what normal controls achieve, may need to be reached to ameliorate metabolic control.

Risk Factors for Cardiovascular Disease

Cardiovascular disease is more prevalent in people with NIDDM (Garcia, McNamara, Gordon, & Kannell, 1974; Robertson & Strong, 1968; Ruderman & Haudenschild, 1984). People with Type II diabetes have two to three times the risk of coronary artery disease as healthy people, an increase associated with abnormalities in both glucose and lipid metabolism. Although glucose intolerance and plasma lipoproteins are abnormal in NIDDM, hyperinsulinemia and insulin resistance may also be atherogenic agents because of their independent association in predicting risk for coronary heart disease (CHD) (Pyorala, 1979). In addition, coagulation factors may play a role in the increased risk for CHD.

Physical training may help prevent the development of atherosclerotic vascular disease (Bjorntorp et al., 1972; Schneider, Vitug, & Ruderman, 1986). Verity and Ismail (1989) report that a short-term exercise training program improves blood lipid profiles in older women with Type II diabetes, yet a 2-year exercise training program did not alter lipids in men of a similar age with NIDDM (Skarfors et al., 1987). Increases in HDL cholesterol after a year of outpatient programs of diet and exercise have been reported in Type II subjects (Vanninen et al., 1992). Verity and Ismail found that postmenopausal women with mild NIDDM who followed a 4-month exercise program increased their $\dot{V}O_2$max and decreased cholesterol while maintaining HDL cholesterol levels, even though their body weight and body fat remained unchanged. Barnard, Lattimore, Holly, Cherny, and Pritikin (1982) studied the response of 60 NIDDM patients to an intense program that included exercise and a diet high in complex carbohydrates and fiber and low in fat (Pritikin diet) and reported markedly reduced serum glucose, cholesterol, and triglyceride levels. The effects of 4 months of exercise training on serum lipids, lipoproteins, and lipid-metabolizing enzymes in NIDDM lowered serum LDL cholesterol, increased serum HDL cholesterol, and reduced triglycerides in the short term, with no changes in apoproteins A-1 or B (Rönnemaa, Marniemi, Puukka, & Kuusi, 1988). Schneider, Kim, Khachadurian, and Ruderman (1988) studied coagulation parameters and fibrinolytic activity in patients with NIDDM before and after a 6-week exercise intervention. Measures were taken at rest and after a 30-min bout of exercise performed at 70% to 75% of $\dot{V}O_2$max. Impaired fibrinolytic activity, elevated concentrations of plasma fibrinogen, and an increased prothrombin time were noted at baseline. Before training, individuals with NIDDM showed a reduced increment in fibrinolysis after acute exercise as compared with nondiabetic controls. Following the exercise training period, no differences were found in plasma fibrinogen levels or exercise-induced increments in fibrinolytic activity, but resting and postexercise-activated partial thromboplastin time and resting fibrinolytic activity were improved in those with NIDDM.

Weight Reduction

Obesity has been shown to be a major characteristic of those with NIDDM (Holbrook et al., 1989; Wing, 1989). Android, or the central pattern of obesity (an increase in intraabdominal fat), is associated with the hyperinsulinemic syndromes of Type II diabetes (Bergstrom et al., 1990; Kissebah et al., 1982). Hyperinsulinemia, insulin resistance, hypertension, dislipoproteinemias, and atherosclerosis are linked in the adult obese individual (Christlieb, Krolewski, Warram, & Soeldner, 1985; Modan et al., 1985; Stout, 1985). Exercise training alone may not improve glycemic control or insulin resistance, especially if obesity is present (Lampman & Schteingart, 1991). Weight reduction for the overweight person with NIDDM reduces blood glucose levels and increases insulin sensitivity (Olefsky, Reaven, & Farquhar, 1974). This therapeutic approach alone may not always be successful, especially if weight reduction is to be achieved (Dahlkoetter, Callahan, & Linton, 1979; Harris & Hallbauer, 1973; Stalonas, Johnson, & Christ, 1987; Wing et al., 1988). When obesity is present a more optimal approach may combine exercise training and caloric restriction (Lampman et al., 1987). Exercise training in combination with a weight reduction diet greatly enhanced glucose disposal rate in Type II diabetics, primarily as a result of an increased rate of nonoxidative carbohydrate storage (Bogardus et al., 1984). In this study, both exercise training and diet and diet alone had similar effects in reducing basal and insulin-suppressed hepatic glucose output. The training group that used diet plus exercise showed a marked improvement in total glucose disposal during the euglycemic clamp test, whereas no change in this measure was observed for the group that used diet alone. A recent study by Segal, Blando, Ginsberg-Fellner, and Edano (1992) demonstrated an increase in thermogenesis in Type II diabetic men after an acute exercise bout following a 12-week program of vigorous cycle ergometer training, even though weight remained constant. These results suggest that a long-term routine exercise program should benefit the obese NIDDM patient, despite no change in body weight.

Oral hypoglycemic agents may also be effective adjuvant therapy for those with Type II diabetes. Fifteen obese patients with NIDDM who used insulin underwent a diet and exercise program for 15 weeks (Lucas et al., 1987). The patients lost an average of 22 pounds, and their frequency and duration of physical exercise increased. Glycemic control by week 15 was unchanged, as were blood lipid concentrations. Both fasting plasma glucose and glucose tolerance improved over the next 15 weeks when an oral hypoglycemic agent was administered up to the 24th week. Another beneficial effect, aside from improvements in $\dot{V}O_2$max and obesity index, was that systolic and diastolic blood pressure decreased by about 10 mm of mercury. Serum lipids and glycosylated hemoglobin remained unchanged.

Summary

The mechanisms for many of the findings discussed in this chapter are not fully understood, but they suggest that habitual exercise may favorably influence many of the multifactorial aberrations in glucose and lipid metabolism in people with Type II diabetes. It is evident that additional research is required to advance our understanding of how exercise training may normalize blood glucose concentrations. Some but not all studies have shown the effects of physical training in Type II diabetes to be beneficial in improving glucose tolerance, insulin sensitivity, and blood glucose control. Exercise training may improve the metabolic abnormalities involving the muscular glucose transport system and prevent hyperglycemia and hyperinsulinemia. The intensity at which exercise is performed may be of particular importance in achieving both cardiovascular and metabolic improvements. For this reason, exercise training may be more efficacious when begun in early life and before the occurrence of overt cardiovascular disease. Furthermore, the response to exercise training in patients with Type II diabetes may vary depending on a number of factors, including obesity, the age of the individual, the state of glucose control, and the degree of initial insulin resistance. Recent findings suggest that individuals who are at risk of developing Type II diabetes may be able to actually prevent or delay its onset if they maintain exercise throughout life. Future studies need to be done in humans to fully delineate the benefits of exercise training in individuals with Type II diabetes. Several areas for future research that may prove fruitful include

- specific glucose transporters (Glut 1/Glut 4),
- glucose transporter effects,
- carbohydrate synthesis and oxidation rates,
- carbohydrate storage sites and rates,
- hepatic and peripheral sensitivity to insulin,
- insulin synthesis and secretion rates,
- insulin receptor binding and postreceptor kinetics,
- interaction of carbohydrate and lipid metabolism,
- risk for cardiovascular complications,
- body composition changes, and
- general physical and mental health.

References

Ahlborg, G., Felig, P., Hagenfeldt, L., Hendler, R., & Wahren, J. (1974). Substrate turnover during prolonged exercise in man: Splanchnic and leg metabolism of glucose, free fatty acids and amino acids. *Journal of Clinical Investigation, 53*, 1078-1084.

Allenberg, K., Johansen, K., & Saltin, B. (1988). Skeletal muscle adaptations to physical training in type II (non-insulin-dependent) diabetes mellitus. *Acta Medica Scandinavica, 223*(4), 365-373.

Andersen, P., & Henriksson, J. (1977). Capillary supply of quadriceps femoris muscle of man: Adaptive response to exercise. *Journal of Physiology, 270*, 677-690.

Andréasson, K., Galuska, D., Thörne, A., Sonnenfield, T., & Wallberg-Henriksson, H. (1991). Decreased insulin-stimulated 3-0-methylglucose transport in in vitro incubated muscle strips from Type II diabetic subjects. *Acta Physiologica Scandinavica, 142*(2), 255-260.

Arner, P., Pollare, T., Lithell, H., & Livingston, J.N. (1987). Defective insulin receptor tyrosine in human skeletal muscle in obesity and type 2 (non-insulin-dependent) diabetes mellitus. *Diabetologia, 30*(6), 437-440.

Barnard, R.J., Lattimore, L., Holly, R.G., Cherny, S., & Pritikin, N. (1982). Response of non-insulin-dependent diabetic patients to an intensive program of diet and exercise. *Diabetes Care, 5*(4), 370-374.

Bergstrom, R.W., Newell-Morris, L.L., Leonetti, D.L., Shuman, W.P., Wahl, P.W., & Fujimoto, W.Y. (1990). Association of elevated fasting C-peptide level and increased intra-abdominal fat distribution with development of NIDDM in Japanese-American men. *Diabetes, 39*, 104-111.

Bjorntorp, P., Fahlen, M., Grimby, G., Gustafson, A., Holm, J., Renstrom, P., & Schersten, T. (1972). Carbohydrate and lipid metabolism in middle-aged physically well trained men. *Metabolism, 21*(11), 1037-1044.

Bjorntorp, P., & Krotkiewski, M. (1985). Exercise treatment in diabetes mellitus. *Acta Medica Scandinavica*, **217**(1), 3-7.

Bogardus, C., Ravussin, E., Robbins, D.C., Wolfe, R.R., Horton, E.S., & Sims, A.H. (1984). Effects of physical training and diet therapy on carbohydrate metabolism in patients with glucose intolerance and non-insulin dependent diabetes mellitus. *Diabetes*, **33**, 311-318.

Bonen, A., Clune, P., & Tan, M.H. (1986). Chronic exercise increases insulin binding in muscles but not liver. *American Journal of Physiology*, **251**, E196-E203.

Bonen, A.B., Tan, M.H., Megeney, L.A., & McDermott, J.C. (1992). Persistence of glucose metabolism after exercise in trained and untrained soleus muscle. *Diabetes Care*, **15**(Suppl. 4), 1694-1700.

Brozinick, J.T., Jr., Etgen, G.J., Jr., Yaspelkis, B.B., III, & Ivy, J.L. (1992). Contraction-activated glucose uptake is normal in insulin-resistant muscle of the obese Zucker rat. *Journal of Applied Physiology*, **73**(1), 382-387.

Burstein, R., Polychronakos, C., Toews, C.J., MacDougall, J.D., Guyda, H.J., & Posner, B.I. (1985). Acute reversal of the enhanced insulin action in trained athletes. Association with insulin receptor changes. *Diabetes*, **34**(8), 756-760.

Caro, J.F., Dohm, L.G., Pories, W.J., & Sinha, M.K. (1989). Cellular alterations in liver, skeletal muscle, and adipose tissue responsible for insulin resistance in obesity and type II diabetes. *Diabetes/Metabolism Reviews*, **5**(8), 665-689.

Caro, J.F., Sinha, M.K., Raju, S.M., Ittoop, O., Pories, W.J., Flickinger, E.G., Meelheim, D., & Dohm, G.L. (1987). Insulin receptor kinase in human skeletal muscle from obese subjects with and without non-insulin-dependent diabetes. *Journal of Clinical Investigation*, **79**(5), 1330-1337.

Christlieb, A.K., Krolewski, A.S., Warram, J.H., & Soeldner, J.S. (1985). Is insulin the link between obesity and hypertension? *Hypertension*, **7**(Suppl. 2), 54-57.

Cortez, M.Y., Torgan, C.E., Brozinick, J.T., Jr., & Ivy, J.L. (1991). Insulin resistance of obese Zucker rats exercise trained at two different intensities. *American Journal of Physiology*, **261**(5 Pt. 1), E613-E619.

Craig, W.B., Garthwaite, S.M., Holloszy, J.O. (1987). Adipocyte insulin resistance: Effects of aging, obesity, exercise, and food restriction. *Journal of Applied Physiology*, **62**(1), 95-100.

Crettaz, M., Horton, E.S., Warzala, L.J., Horton, E.D., & Jeanrenaud, B. (1983). Physical training of Zucker rats: Lack of alleviation of muscle insulin resistance. *American Journal of Physiology*, **244**(4), E414-E420.

Dahlkoetter, J., Callahan, E.J., & Linton, J. (1979). Obesity and the unbalanced energy equation: Exercise vs. eating habit change. *Journal of Consulting and Clinical Psychology*, **47**(5), 898-905.

Davis, T.A., Klahr, S., Tegtmeyer, E.D., Osborne, D.F., Howard, T.L., & Karl, I.E. (1986). Glucose metabolism in epitrochlearis muscle of acutely exercised and trained rats. *American Journal of Physiology*, **250**, E137-E143.

DeFronzo, R.A. (1988). The triumvirate B-cell, muscle and liver: A collusion responsible for NIDDM. *Diabetes, 37*, 667-687.

Douen, A.G., Ramlal, T., Cartee, G.D., & Klip, A. (1990). Exercise modulates the insulin-induced translocation of glucose transporters in rat skeletal muscle. *Federation of European Biochemical Societies Letters,* **26:261**(2), 256-260.

Douen, A.G., Ramlal, T., Rastogi, S., Bilan, P.J., Cartee, G.D., Vranic, M., Holloszy, J.O., & Klip, A. (1990). Exercise induces recruitment of the "insulin-responsive glucose transporter." Evidence for distinct intracellular insulin- and exercise-recruitable transporter pools in skeletal muscle. *Journal of Biological Chemistry,* **15:265**(23), 13427-13430.

Friedman, J.E., Sherman, W.M., Reed, M.J., Elton, C.W., & Dohm, G.L., (1990). Exercise training increases glucose transporter protein GLUT-4 in skeletal muscle of obese Zucker (fa/fa) rats. *Federation of European Biochemical Societies Letters,* **30:268**(1), 13-16.

Garcia, M.J., McNamara, P.M., Gordon, T., & Kannell, W.B. (1974). Morbidity and mortality in diabetics in the Framingham population: Sixteen year follow-up study. *Diabetes, 23*, 105-111.

Harris, M.B., & Hallbauer, E.S. (1973). Self-directed weight control through eating and exercise. *Behavioral Research Therapy,* **11**, 523-529.

Heath, G.W., Gavin, J.R., III., Hinderliter, J.M., Hagberg, J.M., Bloomfield, S.A., & Holloszy, J.O. (1983). Effects of exercise and lack of exercise on glucose tolerance and insulin sensitivity. *Journal of Applied Physiology,* **55**, 512-517.

Henriksson, J., & Reitman, J.S. (1977). Time course of changes in human skeletal muscle succinate dehydrogenase and cytochrome oxidase activities and maximal oxygen uptake with physical activity and inactivity. *Acta Physiologica Scandinavica,* **99**, 91-97.

Holbrook, T.L., Barrett-Connor, E., & Wingard, D.L. (1989). The association of lifetime weight and weight control patterns with diabetes among men and women in an adult community. *International Journal of Obesity,* **13**, 723-729.

Holloszy, J.O., Schultz, J., Kusnierkiewicz, J., Hagberg, J.M., & Ehsani, A.A. (1986). Effects of exercise on glucose tolerance and insulin resistance. Brief review and some preliminary results. *Acta Medica Scandinavica Suppl.,* **711**, 55-65.

Horton, E.S. (1988). Role and management of exercise in diabetes mellitus. *Diabetes Care,* **11**(2), 201-211.

Horton, E.S. (1988). Exercise and diabetes mellitus. *Medical Clinics of North America,* **72**(6), 1301-1321.

Huh, K.B., Park, H.S., Kim, H.M., Lim, S.K., Kim, K.R., & Lee, H.C. (1986). The effects of diet and exercise in the treatment of non-insulin dependent diabetes mellitus. *Korean Journal of Internal Medicine,* **1**(2), 198-204.

Ivy, J.L., Brozinick, J.T., Jr., Torgan, C.E., & Kastello, G.M. (1989). Skeletal muscle glucose transport in obese Zucker rats after exercise training. *Journal of Applied Physiology*, **66**(6), 2635-2641.

Ivy, J.L., Sherman, W.M., Cutler, C.L., & Katz, A.L. (1986). Exercise and diet reduce muscle insulin resistance in obese Zucker rats. *American Journal of Physiology*, **251**, E299-E305.

Ivy, J.L., Young, J.C., McLane, J.A., Fell, R.D., & Holloszy, J.O. (1983). Exercise training and glucose uptake by skeletal muscle in rats. *Journal of Applied Physiology*, **55**(5), 1393-1396.

James, D.E., Burleigh, K.M., Storlien, L.H., Bennett, S.P., & Kraegen, E.W. (1986). Heterogeneity of insulin action in muscle: Influence of blood flow. *American Journal of Physiology*, **251**(4 Pt. 1), E422-E430.

James, D.E., Kraegen, E.W., & Chisholm, D.J. (1985). Effects of exercise training on in vivo insulin action in individual tissues of the rat. *Journal of Clinical Investigation*, **76**(2), 657-666.

Kahn, B.B., Charron, M.J., Lodish, H.F., Cushman, S.W., & Flier, J.S. (1989). Differential regulation of two glucose transporters in adipose cells from diabetic and insulin treated diabetic rats. *Journal of Clinical Investigation*, **84**, 404-411.

Kissebah, A.H., Vydelingum, N., Murray, R., Evans, D.J., Hartz, A.J., Kalkhoff, R.K., & Adams, P.W. (1982). Relation of body fat distribution to metabolic complications of obesity. *Journal of Clinical Endocrinology and Metabolism*, **54**, 254-260.

Koivisto, V.A., & DeFronzo, R.A. (1984). Exercise in the treatment of Type II diabetes. *Acta Endocrinologica*, **262**(Suppl.), 107-111.

Koivisto, V.A., Yki-Jarvinen, H., & DeFronzo, R.A. (1986). Physical training and insulin sensitivity. *Diabetes/Metabolism Reviews*, **1**(4), 445-481.

Krotkiewski, M., Lönnroth, P., Manrwoukas, K., Wroblewski, Z., Rebuffe-Scrive, M., Holme, G., Smith, U., & Bjorntorp, P. (1985). The effects of physical training on insulin secretion and effectiveness and on glucose metabolism in obesity and type 2 (non-insulin-dependent) diabetes mellitus. *Diabetologia*, **28**, 881-890.

Lampman, R.M., Santinga, J.T., Savage, P.J., Bassett, D.R., Hydrick, C.R., Flora, J.D., & Block, W.D. (1985). Effect of exercise training on glucose tolerance, in vivo insulin sensitivity, lipid and lipoprotein concentrations in middle-aged men with mild hypertriglyceridemia. *Metabolism*, **34**(3), 205-211.

Lampman, R.M., & Schteingart, D.E. (1991). Effects of exercise on glucose control, lipid metabolism, and insulin sensitivity in hypertriglyceridemia and non-insulin dependent diabetes mellitus. *Medicine and Science in Sports and Exercise*, **23**(6), 703-712.

Lampman, R.M., Schteingart, D.E., Santinga, J.T., Savage, P.J., Hydrick, C.R., Bassett, D.R., & Block, W.D. (1987). The influence of physical training on glucose tolerance, insulin sensitivity, and lipid and lipoprotein concentrations in middle-aged hypertriglyceridemia, carbohydrate intolerant men. *Diabetologia, 30,* 380-385.

Lillioja, S., Young, A.A., Culter, C.L., Ivy, J.L., Abbott, W.G., Zawadzki, J.K., Yki-Jarvinen, H., Christin, L., Secomb, T.W., & Bogardus, C. (1987). Skeletal muscle capillary density and fiber type are possible determinants of in vivo insulin resistance in man. *Journal of Clinical Investigation, 80*(2), 415-424.

Lithell, H., Krotkiewski, M., Kiens, B., Wroblewski, Z., Holm, G., Stromblad, G., Grimby, G., & Bjorntorp, P. (1985). Non-response of muscle capillary density and lipoprotein-lipase activity to regular training in diabetic patients. *Diabetes Research, 2*(1), 17-21.

Lucas, C.P., Patton, S., Stepke, T., Kinhal, V., Darga, L.L., Carroll-Michals, L., Spafford, T.R., & Kasim, S. (1987). Achieving therapeutic goals in insulin-using diabetic patients with non-insulin-dependent diabetes mellitus. A weight reduction-exercise oral agent approach. *American Journal of Medicine, 18:83*(3A), 3-9.

Mandarino, L., Consoli, A., Thorne, R., & Kelley, D. (1988). Effect of hyperglycemia on oxidative and nonoxidative glucose metabolism in noninsulin-dependent diabetes mellitus (NIDDM): Role of pyruvate dehydrogenase and glycogen synthase. *Diabetes, 37*(Suppl. 1), 77A.

Michel, G., Vocke, T., Flehn, W., Weicker, H., Schwartz, W., & Bieger, W.P. (1984). Bidirectional alteration of insulin receptor affinity by different forms of physical exercise. *American Journal of Physiology, 246,* E153-E159.

Mikines, K.J., Sonne, B., Farrell, P.A., Tronier, B., & Galbo, H. (1988). Effect of physical exercise on sensitivity and responsiveness to insulin in humans. *American Journal of Physiology, 254,* E248-E259.

Minuk, H.L., Vranic, M., Marliss, E.B., Hanna, A.K., Albisser, A.M., & Zinman, B. (1981). Glucoregulatory and metabolic response to exercise in obese non-insulin-dependent diabetes. *American Journal of Physiology, 240,* E458-E464.

Modan, M., Halkin, H., Almog, S., Lusky, A., Eshkol, A., Shefi, M., Shitrit, A., & Fuchs, Z. (1985). Hyperinsulinemia: A link between hypertension, obesity and glucose intolerance. *Journal of Clinical Investigation, 75,* 809-817.

Mondon, C.E., Dolkas, C.B., & Reaven, G.M. (1980). Effects of exercise training on in vivo insulin action in individual tissues of the rat. *Journal of Clinical Investigation, 76,* 657-666.

National Institutes of Health. (1987). Consensus development conference on diet and exercise in non-insulin-dependent diabetes mellitus. *Diabetes Care, 10,* 639-644.

Obermaier-Kusser, B., White, M.F., Pongratz, D.E., Su, Z., & Ermel, B. (1989). A defective intramolecular autoactivation cascade may cause the reduced kinase activity of the skeletal muscle insulin receptor from patients with non-insulin-dependent diabetes mellitus. *Journal of Biological Chemistry, 264*(16), 9497-9504.

Olefsky, J., Reaven, G.M., & Farquhar, J.W. (1974). Effect of weight reduction on obesity: Studies of lipid and carbohydrate metabolism in normal and hyperlipoproteinemic subjects. *Journal of Clinical Investigation, 53*(1), 64-76.

Pedersen, O., Bak, J.F., Anderson, P.H., Lund, S., Moller, D.E., Flier, J.S., & Kahn, B.B. (1990). Evidence against altered expression of GLUT1 or GLUT4 in skeletal muscle of patients with obesity or NIDDM. *Diabetes, 39*(7), 865-870.

Pyorala, K. (1979). Relationship of glucose tolerance and plasma insulin to the incidence of coronary heart disease: Results from two population studies in Finland. *Diabetes Care, 2*(2), 131-141.

Reitman, J.S., Vasquez, B., Klimes, I., & Nagulesparan, M. (1984). Improvement of glucose homeostasis after exercise training in non-insulin-dependent diabetes. *Diabetes Care, 7*(5), 434-441.

Robertson, W.B., & Strong, J.P. (1968). Atherosclerosis in persons with hypertension and diabetes mellitus. *Laboratory Investigation, 18,* 538-551.

Rodnick, K.J., Haskell, W.L., Swislocki, A.L., Foley, J.E., & Reaven, G.M. (1987). Improved insulin action in muscle, liver, and adipose tissue in physically trained human subjects. *American Journal of Physiology, 253,* E489-E495.

Rogers, M.A., Yamamoto, C., King, D.S., Hagberg, J.M., Ehsani, A.A., & Holloszy, J.O. (1988). Improvement in glucose intolerance after 1 wk of exercise in patients with mild NIDDM. *Diabetes Care, 11*(8), 613-618.

Rönnemaa, T., Mattila, K., Lehtonen, A., & Kallio, V. (1986). A controlled randomized study of the effect of long-term physical exercise on the metabolic control in type 2 diabetic patients. *Acta Medica Scandinavica, 220*(3), 219-224.

Rönnemaa, T., Marniemi, J., Puukka, P., & Kuusi, T. (1988). Effects of long-term physical exercise on serum lipids, lipoproteins and lipid metabolizing enzymes in type 2 (non-insulin-dependent) diabetic patients. *Diabetes Research, 7*(2), 79-84.

Ruderman, N.B., Ganda, O.M.P., & Johansen, K. (1979). The effect of physical training on glucose tolerance and plasma lipids in maturity-onset diabetes. *Diabetes, 28*(Suppl.), 89-92.

Ruderman, N.B., & Haudenschild, C. (1984). Diabetes as an atherogenic factor. *Progress in Cardiovascular Diseases, 26,* 373-412.

Saltin, B., Lindgarde, F., Houston, M., Horlin, R., Nygaard, E., & Gad, P. (1979). Physical training and glucose tolerance in middle-aged men with chemical diabetes. *Diabetes, 28*(Suppl. 1), 30-32.

Schneider, S.H., Amorosa, L.F., Khachadurian, A.K., & Ruderman, N.B. (1984). Studies on the mechanism of improved glucose control during regular exercise in type 2 (non-insulin-dependent) diabetes. *Diabetologia, 26*(5), 355-360.

Schneider, S.H., Kim, H.C., Khachadurian, A.K., & Ruderman, N.B. (1988). Impaired fibrinolytic response to exercise in type II diabetes: Effects of exercise and physical training. *Metabolism, 37*(10), 924-929.

Schneider, S.H., Vitug, A., Ruderman, N. (1986). Atherosclerosis and physical activity. *Diabetes/Metabolism Reviews, 1*(4), 513-553.

Schteingart, D.E., Lampman, R.M., & Starkman, M.N. (1985). Effects of exercise during weight reduction in severe obesity. *International Journal of Obesity, 9*, A92.

Segal, K.R., Blando, L., Ginsberg-Fellner, F., & Edano, A. (1992). Postprandial thermogenesis at rest and postexercise before and after physical training in lean, obese, and mildly diabetic men. *Metabolism, 41*(8), 868-878.

Segal, K.R., Edano, A., Abalos, A., Albu, J., Blando, L., Tomas, M.B., & Pi-Sunyer, F.X. (1991). Effect of exercise training on insulin sensitivity and glucose metabolism in lean, obese, and diabetic men. *Journal of Applied Physiology, 71*(6), 2402-2411.

Sherman, W.M., Katz, A.L., Cutler, C.L., Withers, R.T., & Ivy, J.L. (1988). Glucose transport: Locus of muscle insulin resistance in obese Zucker rats. *American Journal of Physiology, 255*(3 Pt. 1), E374-E382.

Skarfors, E.T., Wegener, T.A., Lithel, H., & Selinus, I. (1987). Physical training as treatment for type II (non-insulin-dependent) diabetes in elderly men: A feasibility study over 2 years. *Diabetologia, 30*(12), 930-933.

Soman, V.R., Koivisto, V.A., Deibert, D., Felig, P., & DeFronzo, R.A. (1979). Increased insulin sensitivity and insulin binding to monocytes after physical training. *New England Journal of Medicine, 29:301*(22), 1200-1204.

Stalonas, P.M., Johnson, W.G., & Christ, M. (1987). Behaviour modification for obesity: The evaluation of exercise, contingency management, and programme adherence. *Journal of Consulting and Clinical Psychology, 46*, 463-469.

Stout, R.W. (1985). Overview of the association between insulin and atherosclerosis. *Metabolism, 34*(Suppl. 1), 7-12.

Tan, M.H., & Bonen, A. (1987). Effects of physical training on insulin binding and glucose uptake in mouse soleus muscle. *Canadian Journal of Physiology and Pharmacology, 65*, 2231-2234.

Taylor, R., Ram, P., Zimmet, P., Raper, L.R., & Ringrose, H. (1984). Physical activity and prevalence of diabetes in Melanesian and Indian men in Fiji. *Diabetologia, 27*(6), 578-582.

Taylor, S.I., Kadowaki, T., Kadowaki, H., Accili, D., Cama, A., & McKeon, C. (1990). Mutations in insulin-receptor gene in insulin-resistant patients. *Diabetes Care, 13*, 257-279.

Torgan, C.E., Brozinick, J.T., Jr., Kastello, G.M., & Ivy, J.L. (1989). Muscle morphological and biochemical adaptations to training in obese Zucker rats. *Journal of Applied Physiology, 67*(5), 1807-1813.

Trovati, M., Carta, Q., Cavalot, F., Vitali, S., Banaudi, C., Lucchina, P.G., Fiocchi, F., Emanuelli, G., & Lenti, G. (1984). Influence of physical training on blood glucose control, glucose tolerance, insulin secretion, and insulin action in non-insulin-dependent diabetic patients. *Diabetes Care,* **7**(5), 416-420.

Unger, R.H., & Grundy, S. (1985). Hyperglycemia as an inducer as well as a consequence of impaired islet function and insulin resistance. *Diabetologia,* **28**, 119-121.

Vallerand, A.L., Lupien, J., & Bukowlecki, L.J. (1986). Synergistic improvement of glucose tolerance by sucrose feeding and exercise training. *American Journal of Physiology,* **259**, E607-E614.

Vallerand, A.L., Lupien, J., Deshaies, Y., & Bukowieki, L.J. (1986). Intensive exercise training does not improve intravenous glucose tolerance in severely diabetic rats. *Hormone and Metabolic Research,* **18**(2), 79-81.

Vanninen, E., Uusitupa, M., Siitonen, O., Laitinen, J., & Länsimies, E. (1992). Habitual physical activity, aerobic capacity and metabolic control in patients with newly-diagnosed type 2 (non-insulin-dependent) diabetes mellitus: Effect of 1-year diet and exercise intervention. *Diabetologia,* **35**, 340-346.

Verity, L.S., & Ismail, A.H. (1989). Effects of exercise on cardiovascular disease risk in women with NIDDM. *Diabetes Research and Clinical Practice,* **6**(1), 27-35.

Vinten, J. Norgaad-Peterson, L., Sonne, B., & Galbo, H. (1985). Effect of physical training on glucose transporters in fat cell fractions. *Biochemica Biophysica Acta,* **16:841**, 223-227.

Wahren, J., Felig, P., Ahlborg, G., & Jorfeldt, L. (1971). Glucose metabolism during leg exercise in men. *Journal of Clinical Investigation,* **50**, 2715-2725.

Wallberg-Henrikkson, H. (1986). Repeated exercise regulates glucose transport capacity in skeletal muscle. *Acta Physiologica Scandinavica,* **127**, 39-43.

Wardzala, L.J., Crettaz, M., Horton, E.D., Jeanrenaud, B., & Horton, E.S. (1982). Physical training of lean and genetically obese Zucker rats: Effect on fat cell metabolism. *American Journal of Physiology,* **243**(5), E418-E426.

Wing, R.R. (1989). Behavioral strategies for weight reduction in obese type II diabetic patients. *Diabetics Care,* **12**(2), 139-144.

Wing, R.R., Epstein, L.H., Paternostro-Bayles, M., Kriska, A., Nowalk, M.P., & Gooding, W. (1988). Exercise in a behavioural weight control programme for obese patients with type 2 (non-insulin-dependent) diabetes. *Diabetologia,* **31**(12), 902-909.

Yki-Jarvinen, H., & Koivisto, V. (1983). Effects of body composition on insulin sensitivity. *Diabetes,* **32**, 965-969.

Young, J.C., Enslin, J., & Kuca, B. (1989). Exercise intensity and glucose tolerance in trained and nontrained subjects. *Journal of Applied Physiology,* **67**, 39-43.

Chapter 6

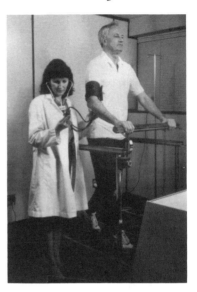

The Clinical Application of Exercise in Type I Diabetes

It is not clearly documented that exercise improves glycemic control in insulin-dependent diabetes mellitus, possibly because increased caloric consumption or decreased insulin treatment is necessary to prevent exercise-associated hypoglycemia. As described in chapter 3, however, regular exercise does diminish insulin resistance, improve glucose metabolism, and reduce cardiovascular disease (CVD) risk. Thus, exercise programs should be designed to assist people with Type I diabetes to exercise safely and to decrease their risk of cardiovascular disease. Little information, however, has been available to professionals on planning and carrying out an individualized exercise "prescription" for patients with diabetes. The purpose of this chapter is to provide basic guidelines and some specific recommendations for designing and implementing clinically safe individualized exercise programs that may benefit patients with diabetes.

It is the role of the clinical management team to provide appropriate information to the patient on exercise. This team is made up of health professionals with areas of specialization: usually a physician specializing in diabetes treatment, a nurse specialist or diabetes educator, a dietitian, and an exercise specialist or exercise physiologist. This chapter provides information on including exercise in the diabetes management plan, which can be applied by any member of the management team.

Before receiving a recommended individual exercise program, each patient must undergo a thorough screening. The first section of this chapter will cover appropriate preexercise screening procedures and the information necessary to obtain from patients before beginning exercise. The next section discusses how to design and implement an exercise program, including glycemic control, recommendations for glucose monitoring, and modifications in diet and insulin therapy. The third section discusses the influence of exercise on the complications of diabetes. It provides specific recommendations for appropriate types of exercise and precautions for patients with neuropathy, retinopathy, and nephropathy. This section also deals with the specifics of exercise programs, including follow-up and the risks and benefits of exercise for these patients. The chapter closes with several case studies. Although some of this information is not backed by extensive research, it has been used clinically with success.

Screening

When seeing a patient for the first time, the professional must answer the question, "Can this individual participate in exercise safely?" By assessing the patient's diabetes and general health and screening for possible underlying complications (Campaigne, 1988), relevant clinical information, including diabetes control, complications associated with diabetes, and the health of the cardiovascular system and other systems, can be obtained. Specific recommended screening procedures for patients prior to beginning an exercise program are outlined in Table 6.1. Patients with long-standing diabetes (more than 10 years) are at a much greater risk of developing underlying complications. It is, therefore, important to assess these individuals carefully before recommending exercise. Changes in blood pressure and other hemodynamics during exercise increase the risk of small vessel damage for patients with long-standing diabetes.

In addition to patients with long disease duration, those with renal disease and those over 35 years of age are at an increased risk of coronary artery disease. These individuals should be carefully examined for cardiovascular disease and should undergo a graded exercise test before exercise is recommended.

Patients at high risk for underlying cardiovascular disease include

- those with diabetes of long duration (more than 10 years),
- those with renal disease, and
- those who are over 35 years of age.

The patient's private physician should be asked to provide specific evaluations (Table 6.1) that are required before the patient begins exercise.

Table 6.1   Recommended Screening Procedures

History and physical examination
(for patients newly diagnosed or without up-to-date records)
a. Review all systems
b. Identification of medical problems (e.g., asthma, arthritis)
Diabetes evaluation

a. Glycosylated hemoglobin (HbA$_1$)
b. Ophthalmoscopic exam (retinopathy)
c. Neurologic exam (neuropathy)
d. Nephrologic evaluation (microalbumin or protein in urine)
e. Nutritional status evaluation (underweight/overweight)
Cardiovascular evaluation

a. Blood pressure
b. Peripheral pulses
c. Bruits
d. 12-lead electrocardiogram
e. Serum lipid profile (total cholesterol, triglycerides, HDL and LDL cholesterol)
f. Graded exercise test (those over 35 years of age or suspected history of or documented CHD or multiple CHD risk factors present or diabetes of longer than 10 years)

Note. The graded exercise test should be performed according to the guidelines of the American College of Sports Medicine.

Table 6.1 provides recommendations; however, if the physician orders more or fewer screening examinations, the order should be complied with. Both the evaluation of the patient's diabetes and the cardiovascular examination should be used to develop an individualized exercise program. Any other medical problems (e.g., asthma, arthritis) should be taken into consideration when developing the program.

Absolute contraindications for strenuous exercise include

- poor glycemic control (see Table 6.2),
- proliferative retinopathy,
- *microangiopathy*,
- neuropathy,
- nephropathy, and
- evidence of cardiovascular disease.

Design and Implementation of the Exercise Program

Whenever possible, the exercise program should be designed with the physician. This provides time for a positive interaction between the

Table 6.2   General Guidelines for Making Food Adjustments for Exercise

Type of exercise and examples:	If blood glucose is:	Increase food intake by:	Suggestions of food to use:
Exercise of short duration and/or low to moderate intensity	80-100 mg/dl	10 to 15 g of carbohydrate per hr	1 fruit or 1 bread exchange
Examples: Walking a half mile or leisurely bicycling for less than 30 min	above 100 mg/dl	Not necessary to increase food	
Exercise of moderate intensity	80-100 mg/dl	25 to 50 g of carbohydrate before exercise; then 10 to 15 g per hr of exercise, if needed	1/2 meat sandwich with a low fat milk or fruit exchange
Examples: tennis, swimming, jogging, leisurely bicycling, gardening, golfing, or vacuuming for 1 hr	100-180 mg/dl	10 to 15 g of carbohydrate per hr of exercise	1 fruit or 1 bread exchange
	180-250 mg/dl	Not necessary to increase food	
	250 mg/dl or greater	Don't begin exercise until blood glucose is under 250 mg/dl	

Strenuous activity			
Examples: football, hockey, racquetball or soccer, running, strenuous bicycling or swimming, shoveling heavy snow	80-100 mg/dl	50 g of carbohydrate; monitor blood glucose carefully	1 meat sandwich (2 slices of bread) with a fruit exchange; 1/2 meat sandwich with a low fat milk or fruit exchange
	180-250 mg/dl	10 to 15 g of carbohydrate per hr of exercise	1 fruit or 1 bread exchange
	above 250 mg/dl	Exercise should not take place unless blood glucose less than 250 mg/dl	

From *Learning to Live Well With Diabetes* (p. 58) by D.D. Etzwiler, M.J. Franz, P. Hollander, and J.O. Joynes, 1987, Minnetonka, MN: Chronimed Publishing, Inc. Copyright 1987 by International Diabetes Center, Park Nicollet Medical Center. Adapted by permission.

members of the management team, the physician, and the patient. If this interaction takes place during the design of the program, everyone will clearly understand goals and expectations, which can then be reinforced in subsequent meetings with the physician and individual members of the management team.

If patients are contraindicated for specific types of exercise (e.g., because of peripheral neuropathy resulting in insensitive feet), they should be given careful guidance in activities that are most appropriate (e.g., swimming or cycling).

Risks and Benefits of Exercise

The patient should be informed about the risks and benefits of exercise. If a thorough screening examination is performed and a trained specialist prescribes an exercise program based on the screening, the risks of regular physical activity are minimal. Risks may include fatigue and muscle soreness during the early stages of an exercise program. The patient should be instructed on how to warm up and cool down, stretch, and alter the program's intensity or duration when necessary. The occurrence of hypoglycemia is the risk for patients participating in exercise; they should be counseled on how to avoid hypoglycemia during and after exercise (Table 6.3). Table 6.4 gives the risks and benefits of exercise for patients

Table 6.3   General Guidelines for Avoiding Hypoglycemia During and After Exercise

Blood glucose monitoring
1. Monitor blood glucose immediately before, during (every 30 min) and 15 min after exercise.
2. Delay exercise if blood glucose is 250 mg/dl or higher or ketones are present.
3. Consume carbohydrates if blood glucose is ≤ 80-100 mg/dl.
4. Learn individual glucose response to different types of exercise.
5. Avoid exercising late at night.

Insulin
1. Decrease insulin dose:
   a. Intermediate-acting insulin: Decrease by 30% to 35% on the day of exercise.
   b. Intermediate- and short-acting insulin: Omit dose of short-acting insulin that precedes exercise.
   c. Multiple doses of short-acting insulin: Reduce the dose prior to exercise by 30% to 35% and supplement carbohydrates.
   d. Continuous subcutaneous infusion: Eliminate mealtime bolus or increment that precedes or immediately follows exercise.
2. Avoid exercising muscle underlying injections of short-acting insulin for 1 hr after injection.
3. Do not exercise at the time of peak insulin action.

From "Exercise and Type I Diabetes Mellitus" by J.A. Vitung, S.H. Schneider, and N.B. Ruderman. In *Exercise and Sport Sciences Reviews* (Vol. 16) (pp. 285-304) by K. Pandolf (Ed.), 1988, New York: McGraw-Hill, Inc. Copyright 1988 by McGraw-Hill Inc. Adapted by permission.

Table 6.4   Risks and Benefits of Exercise for Patients With Type I Diabetes

Risks		Benefits
Symptoms	Treatment	
Fatigue	Learn to gauge exercise intensity	Improved insulin sensitivity
Muscle soreness	Learn stretching and warm up techniques	Improved blood lipids, decreased TG, increased HDL/TC, decreased LDL-C
Hypoglycemia	Increase caloric intake; reduce insulin dose	
Hyperglycemia	Reduce exercise intensity	Maintenance or loss of body weight, decreased body fat, possible increased lean body mass
Aggravation of existing complications	Careful screening, exercise prescription, and regular evaluation by diabetes management team	Improved physical fitness level
		Improved blood pressure (if initially elevated)
		Prevent CV decline from disuse when complications are present
		Improved self-esteem and sense of well-being

with Type I diabetes. The benefits of exercise should be discussed. They include improved insulin sensitivity, improved blood lipid profiles, decreased heart rate and blood pressure at rest, decreased body weight, maintenance of lean body mass with weight reduction, and possible decreased risk of the premature morbidity and mortality of coronary heart disease.

Patients should not be led to believe that exercise will improve glycemic control, as most research has not documented improvements in glycemic control. However, it is possible that insulin requirements may be decreased. In addition, improved self-esteem and self-confidence should aid in developing the patient's optimal diabetes management habits. Table 6.5 lists some special precautions that should be given to the patient beginning an exercise program.

Glycemic Control.   Assessment of glycemic control is of extreme importance in the management of individuals with diabetes. This aspect of diabetes care needs reemphasis when initiating exercise for these patients.

Table 6.5   Special Precautions When Recommending Exercise for Patients With Insulin-Dependent Diabetes

Complication	Precaution
Retinopathy[1,2]	Avoid strenuous, high-intensity activities that involve breath holding (e.g., weight lifting and isometrics). Avoid activities that lower the head (e.g., yoga, gymnastics) or that risk jarring the head.
Hypertension	Avoid heavy weight lifting or holding breath. Perform primarily dynamic exercise using large muscle groups, such as walking and cycling at a moderate intensity.
Autonomic neuropathy[2]	Likelihood of hypoglycemia and hypertension. Elevated resting heart rate and reduced maximal heart rate. Use of RPE[3] recommended. Prone to dehydration and hypothermia.
Peripheral neuropathy	Avoid exercise that may cause trauma to the feet (e.g., prolonged hiking, jogging, or walking on uneven surfaces). Nonweight-bearing activities are most appropriate (e.g., cycling and swimming). Regular assessment of the feet recommended. The feet should be kept clean and dry. Careful choice of shoes for proper fit.
Nephropathy	Avoid exercise that raises blood pressure (e.g., weight lifting, high-intensity aerobic exercises, and breath holding).
All patients	Carry identification with diabetes information. Rehydrate carefully (drink fluids before, during, and after exercise). Avoid exercise in the heat of the day and in direct sunlight (wear hat and suncreen when in sun).

1. If proliferative retinopathy is present and the patient has recently undergone photocoagulation or surgical treatment or is not properly treated, exercise is contraindicated.
2. Submaximal exercise testing recommended for patients with proliferative retinopathy and autonomic neuropathy.
3. RPE = Rate of Perceived Exertion.

As discussed in chapter 2, exercise can profoundly influence blood glucose levels, and in turn blood glucose can affect the metabolic response to exercise. Several areas of importance for good glycemic control include

- careful glucose monitoring,
- dietary management and intake, and
- management of the mode and amount of insulin therapy.

Glucose Monitoring,   Close blood glucose monitoring should be encouraged for patients beginning an exercise program, as each may react differently to changes in their treatment plan. Patients should be instructed to monitor their own blood glucose levels according to Table 6.3. When starting an exercise program, blood glucose levels should be checked before exercise, as often as every 15 min during exercise (less frequently for more experienced patients), immediately after exercise, and 4 to 5 hrs following exercise to determine if and when to alter the treatment plan to maintain near-normal blood glucose levels and avoid episodes of either hypoglycemia or hyperglycemia. In addition, assessing glucose control is important before each exercise session to check for elevated blood glucose levels. If severe hyperglycemia (blood glucose greater than or equal to 250 mg/dl), ketones, or both are present, the individual should refrain from exercise until normoglycemia is achieved (Table 6.3). Low-intensity exercise is recommended when blood glucose is elevated (180 mg/dl to 250 mg/dl).

Some individuals have reported hypoglycemic reactions 24 to 48 hr after exercise, probably related to a depletion of carbohydrate stores, increases in insulin sensitivity, or both. Based on carefully obtained blood glucose records, appropriate modifications in diet and insulin can be recommended (Tables 6.2 and 6.3). When exercise is of a consistent intensity and duration and is performed at the same time each day, a routine can be developed to prevent hypoglycemia or hyperglycemia.

Diet

A common question asked by patients is how much carbohydrate to consume during exercise to meet their needs. It is difficult to give precise information because of wide individual variations; however, estimates of energy requirements can be given based on the intensity and duration of activity. Table 6.2 gives general guidelines for dietary modifications for exercise of varying intensity and duration. These are general guidelines, and each individual's specific needs will vary. The professional who prescribes exercise for the individual with diabetes should use these general guidelines to write a specific set of recommendations for that individual.

For example, 30 min of moderate-intensity exercise requires approximately 15 to 30 g of carbohydrate. These guidelines are only approximate, and actual carbohydrate requirements will depend on many factors, including

- exercise intensity and duration,
- preceding diet,
- circulating insulin levels,
- individual fitness level, and
- the need for exogenous carbohydrate for maintenance of blood glucose in the normal range.

As mentioned previously, it is particularly helpful to monitor blood glucose during exercise of varying intensity and duration to determine individual responses.

After a prolonged exercise period, the patient may experience hypoglycemic reactions the following day. Substantial amounts of liver and muscle glycogen are utilized during prolonged activity. Glycogen or carbohydrate stores are replenished after exercise, a process that may take up to 24 (sometimes 48) hr. Blood glucose levels may fall during this period because of the preferential use of glucose for replacing glycogen. The professional who prescribes exercise should tell the person with diabetes that foods high in carbohydrates (breads, pasta, juice, etc.) should be eaten soon after the exercise session to prevent hypoglycemia and help restore glycogen levels. Optimally, glycogen reserves should be replaced in the hours immediately following exercise, but patients may need blood glucose monitoring up to 48 hr after prolonged exercise. In healthy subjects, carbohydrates with a high to moderate glycemic index appear to restore glycogen most effectively in the 4 hr immediately after exercise (Coyle, 1993). Foods with a high glycemic index are not generally recommended for those with diabetes; however, with prolonged exercise these foods may be beneficial. This is an area of possible future research.

In the 24 hr after completing exercise sessions of greater intensity or longer duration than usual, an increase in caloric intake is indicated, with absolute increases dependent on the duration of the exercise performed (Table 6.2). Let the patient know that small reductions in insulin dose may also be required, especially when snacking is not possible.

Insulin

Patients may increase their caloric intake to compensate for increased energy expenditure with exercise. Because elevated insulin levels have been shown to be a risk factor for coronary heart disease, reductions in insulin dose prior to exercise may be more appropriate, however (Haffner, Stern, Mazuda, Mitchell, & Patterson, 1990; Stou, 1979). Recommendations for insulin reduction can be made after assessing individual needs, based on the general guidelines for altering insulin dose to prevent hypoglycemia in Table 6.3. The initial insulin levels and the time of day need consideration when exercise is anticipated (Ruegemer et al., 1990). Most insulin regimens may be altered when exercise is planned in advance. Table 6.6 gives the activity characteristics of insulin, and it can be used to design exercise programs for individuals using these types of insulin. Keep in mind that general recommendations on altering the insulin dose will probably need to be altered to fit each individual's situation.

Intermediate-Acting Insulin.   Individuals taking a single dose of intermediate-acting insulin may decrease the dose 30% to 35% in the morning before exercise or they may change to a split dose, taking two thirds of

Table 6.6   Activity Characteristics of Insulins*

	Onset (hr)	Peak (hr)	Duration (hr)
Rapid acting			
Insulin injection (regular)	1/2-1	2-4	5-7
Prompt insulin zinc suspension (Semilente)	1-3	2-8	12-16
Intermediate acting			
Insulin zinc susp. (Lente)	1-3	6-12	24-28
Isophane insulin susp. (NPH)	1-3	6-12	24-28
Long acting			
Extended insulin zinc susp. (Ultralente)	4-6	18-24	36+
Protamine zinc insulin susp. (PZI)	4-6	14-24	36+

*Onset, peak, and duration of action vary considerably and are dependent upon the individual patient, injection site, vascularity, and temperature.

the usual dose in the morning and the remaining one-third dose before dinner, if it is needed after exercise (Horton, 1988). If an individual is taking a combination of intermediate-acting and short-acting insulins, short-acting insulin can be reduced by 50%, or it can be omitted before exercise. Individuals using this type of therapy may choose to decrease the intermediate-acting insulin before exercise and take supplemental short-acting insulin as needed after exercise.

Short-Acting Insulin.   If a patient is on multiple doses of short-acting insulin alone, the preexercise dose may be lowered by 30% to 50%, and doses following exercise may be adjusted based on glucose monitoring. Based on recent findings discussed in chapter 2, pages 45-48, when insulin-infusion is used the basal infusion rate may be decreased during exercise and the bolus before the meal decreased or omitted. If these measures to decrease infusion rates are not taken, hypoglycemia may occur, although this has not been a universal finding (Martin, Robbins, Bergenstal, LaGrange, & Rubenstein, 1982; Schiffrin, Parikh, Marliss, & Desrosiers, 1984). As with subcutaneous insulin injection, careful monitoring of blood glucose and personal experience can be used to adjust exercise and postexercise basal infusion rates to maintain optimal blood glucose levels. When exercise is prolonged, the premeal bolus can be reduced by 50% and the basal infusion stopped during exercise (Sonnenberg, Kemmer, & Berger, 1990). A 25% reduction in the basal infusion rate has been found to reduce the occurrence of hypoglycemia after prolonged exercise (Sonnenberg et al., 1990).

Human Insulin.   The use of human insulin has become more common in recent years. Human, soluble insulin is more rapidly absorbed than porcine insulin under resting conditions (Federlin, Laube, & Velcovsky, 1981; Pramming, Lauritzen, Thorsteinsson, Johansen, & Binder, 1984). The absorption of human insulin during exercise is enhanced significantly over the resting absorption rate; the increase in human insulin absorption, however, was less pronounced ($40 \pm 19\%$ vs. $105 \pm 40\%$) than the absorption of porcine insulin with exercise (Fernqvist, Linde, Ostman, & Gunnarsson, 1986). The effect of lowering blood glucose was similar for both insulins, and subcutaneous blood flow was unaltered by exercise in both groups. Thus, even though human insulin is absorbed more rapidly than porcine insulin under basal conditions, exercise increases absorption of porcine insulin to a greater degree than human insulin and eliminates the resting difference in absorption rate between the two insulins. Using human insulin does not appear to increase the risk of exercise-induced hypoglycemia when compared with porcine insulin.

Site of Insulin Injection.   The site of insulin injection may influence the risk of hypoglycemia. Subcutaneous insulin injection is the most common way to administer insulin in patients with Type I diabetes. Differences in insulin absorption from various sites can negatively influence glycemic control (Binder, Lauritzen, Faber, & Pramming, 1984). The rate of insulin absorption during exercise varies, depending on the site of injection (Berger et al., 1979; Koivisto & Felig, 1978; Koivisto & Felig, 1980; Zinman et al., 1977). Insulin injected into the subcutaneous tissues overlying an exercising muscle is absorbed faster than from a site away from the active muscle mass (Berger et al., 1979; Koivisto & Felig, 1978; Koivisto & Felig, 1980; Zinman et al., 1977; Zinman, Vranic, Albisser, Leibel, & Marliss, 1979). Frid, Ostman, and Linde (1990) have observed that compared with subcutaneous injection, intramuscular injection of insulin in the thigh before leg exercise represents a previously unobserved risk for hypoglycemia in Type I patients. Frid and Linde (1986) demonstrated that accidental intramuscular injection of insulin occurs frequently in Type I patients and is more common when perpendicular injection techniques are used. Frid et al. (1990) demonstrated that the risk of intramuscular injection and resulting hypoglycemia could be minimized by injection into a skinfold or by use of shorter needles when injection is in the thigh. Thus, to prevent accidental intramuscular injection and hypoglycemia, patients should be advised to inject into a skinfold or to use needles less than 8 mm in length for thigh injection, especially before exercise.

Possible ways to prevent exercise-induced hypoglycemia when using insulin injections include these:

- Inject insulin in a nonexercising muscle group.
- Prevent intramuscular injection by
  - avoiding perpendicular injection,
  - injecting into a skinfold, and
  - using needles less than 8 mm long for thigh injection.

Timing and Mode of Insulin Treatment. A variety of times of day may be appropriate to exercise, although a basic recommendation is not exercising at the time of peak insulin action. If one must exercise at a specific time, the insulin dose should be reduced to prevent peak effect at time of exercise (e.g., decrease long-acting insulin to prevent late-afternoon hypoglycemic reactions). Figure 6.1 illustrates a typical mixed-split dose insulin regimen and the patterns of insulin effects on blood glucose throughout the day. In general, exercise should be recommended

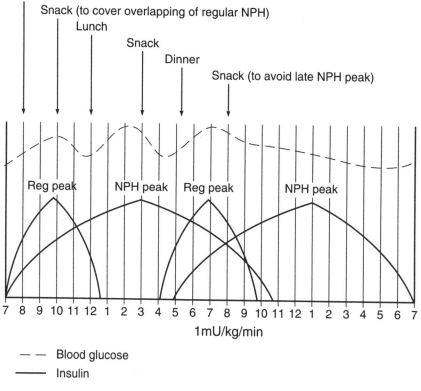

Figure 6.1 Blood glucose and insulin peaks, showing how insulin can help cover the glycemic response to meals and snacks.

From *Learning to Live Well With Diabetes* (p. 137) by D.D. Etzwiler, M.J. Franz, P. Hollander, and J.O. Joynes, 1987, Minnetonka, MN: Chronimed Publishing, Inc. Copyright 1987 by International Diabetes Center, Park Nicollet Medical Center. Adapted by permission.

at times when the insulin effects are lowest and blood glucose is on the rise. To prevent hypoglycemia when exercise is unplanned, a rapidly assimilated carbohydrate snack can be consumed prior to exercise. Exercising before insulin and breakfast may decrease the need for short-acting insulin. Once an exercise schedule is established, insulin dose and caloric intake can be adjusted to optimize glycemic control.

In the case of a runner, if a 10 km race is planned and the individual usually runs 6 to 10 mi per day, no change in insulin would be indicated. For individuals using both long-acting and short-acting insulin, the short-acting insulin should be reduced in accordance with the distance and estimated time of the race. For example, an individual racing at 10:00 a.m. who eats a light breakfast at 7:00 a.m., preceded by insulin injection at 6:45 a.m., would have to reduce short-acting insulin because its peak action is approximately at race time. Smaller doses of insulin may produce a shorter and more rapid peak action. For early morning events of longer duration, it may not be necessary to take insulin at all because, as mentioned, the runner should begin an event with slightly elevated glucose (greater than 140 mg/dl) levels. It is advisable to have the runner consume some rapidly assimilated carbohydrate every 15 to 20 min during competition. Because water is necessary in maintaining hydration and performance, some type of dilute glucose solution (5% to 8%), such as some of the commercially available drinks with glucose polymers, is recommended to help prevent heat exhaustion and hypoglycemia during exercise.

The above adjustments are recommended when exercise is planned, but many individuals will take part in spontaneous exercise at some point. When exercise is not planned in advance, frequent glucose monitoring should be done so adjustments in insulin dose can be made and supplemental feedings given, especially if exercise is prolonged.

Exercise and Complications of Diabetes

Even though exercise is routinely recommended for patients with diabetes, exercise is often neglected when the secondary complications of diabetes occur. Lack of exercise for individuals with secondary complications will decrease functional capacity (Valbona, 1982). Functional changes, both physiological and biochemical, can occur after 3 days of inactivity. Clinical manifestations include decreased physical work capacity, muscle atrophy, negative protein balance, osteoporosis, renal lithiasis, pulmonary and cardiovascular deconditioning, and mental depression, among others (Valbona). The complications of diabetes specifically involve these systems; therefore, the combination of diabetes and disuse leads to greater disability than would diabetes alone (Graham & Lasko-McCarthey, 1990).

Exercise can help prevent or reverse disuse and deterioration of the organ systems for those with diabetes, even in the presence of severe complications, as will be described next.

To recommend clinically sound exercise programs for patients with diabetes, it is extremely important to understand not only the individual needs of the patient but also the complications of diabetes. The clinical management team must consider how exercise can affect and be affected by any underlying complications. Carefully conducted screening should reveal any complications that would influence the exercise recommendations. Some unique concerns for the patient with diabetes that warrant close attention include autonomic and peripheral (sensory) neuropathy, retinopathy, and nephropathy. Most patients with diabetes have some neuropathy after 2 to 3 years duration. The occurrence of neuropathy is associated with glucose control; individuals in poor control are more likely to develop it. Clinical manifestations of neuropathy include both sensory and motor deficits.

Autonomic Neuropathy

Abnormal autonomic function is common among those with diabetes of long duration. These abnormalities have been postulated to interfere with exercise and predispose individuals with them to exercise-induced hypoglycemia. Individuals with visual impairment frequently have cardiovascular autonomic dysfunction and may be prone to the development of hypoglycemia (Bernbaum, Albert, & Cohen, 1989). Abnormalities in autonomic function manifested by abnormal heart rate, blood pressure response, or both could limit the capability to perform exercise (Hilsted, Galbo, & Christensen, 1979, 1980; Hilsted, Galbo, Christensen, Parving, & Benn, 1982; Kahn, Zola, Juni, & Vinik, 1986; Margonata et al., 1986). Hypertension (Karlefors, 1966) and hypotension (Hilsted et al., 1979; Hilsted et al., 1982; Kahn et al., 1986; Margonato et al., 1986) have both been described during exercise in patients with abnormal autonomic function. Exercise tolerance in the person with diabetic autonomic neuropathy may be extremely limited because of impaired sympathetic and parasympathetic nervous systems that normally augment cardiac output and redistribute blood flow to the working muscle.

Noninvasive testing of cardiovascular reflexes to assess autonomic function has been described extensively. Monitoring heart rate and blood pressure response to physiologic maneuvers of postural change and respiratory variation is frequently used to assess the autonomic nervous system (Ewing et al., 1986; Ewing, Martyn, Young, & Clarke, 1985). Heart rate response abnormalities by themselves may be one way to detect mild to moderate dysfunction, whereas abnormal blood pressure response is associated with more severe autonomic dysfunction.

As previously shown, recovery from hypoglycemia is partially mediated through the sympathetic nervous system and may be impaired when autonomic neuropathy is present (Hoeldtke, Boden, Shuman, & Owen, 1982). Bernbaum et al. (1989) assessed the parameters of autonomic dysfunction in diabetic subjects with severe retinopathy in relation to exercise testing results. They found no correlation between the decrease in blood glucose after exercise and cardiac autonomic dysfunction. The amount of regular insulin injected had the highest correlation with a fall in blood glucose. Severe retinopathy of these patients did not interfere with their ability to perform exercise.

Parasympathetic neuropathy has been thought to precede sympathetic neuropathy (Ewing, Campbell, & Clarke, 1981). But results of a study by Bergstrom, Manhem, Bramnert, Lilia and Sundkvist (1989) demonstrated for the first time that sympathetic neuropathy can occur without conventional signs of parasympathetic neuropathy. Bergstrom et al., 1989 showed that patients with Type I diabetes who exhibited abnormal response to standard tests of autonomic neuropathy had an impaired catecholamine response to exercise without signs of parasympathetic neuropathy. Noradrenaline (which Hoeldke and Cilmi [1984] showed to reflect true appearance rate and not impaired clearance in subjects with diabetes) was used as an indicator of sympathetic activity. At a workload of 80% maximum working capacity, the noradrenaline response to exercise was reduced in patients with an abnormal acceleration index (impaired adrenomedullary function) compared with controls, and these patients showed an isolated abnormal break index (impaired parasympathetic function), the latter being a new finding. Thus, exercise testing may be an adjunct means of assessing the extent of autonomic neuropathy in Type I patients. Further work needs to be done in this area.

To summarize, the following are risks for exercise when autonomic neuropathy is present:

• Hypoglycemia
• Abnormal blood pressure response (hypertension and hypotension after vigorous exercise)
• Abnormal heart rate response (increased at rest and decreased maximally)
• Impaired sympathetic and parasympathetic nervous system
• Abnormal thermoregulation (prone to dehydration)

Exercise for Autonomic Neuropathy.   Patients with neuropathy are at high risk for developing complications during exercise. Sudden death and silent myocardial infarction have been attributed to autonomic neuropathy in diabetes in which the heart has become unresponsive to nerve impulses (Ewing & Clark, 1982). This can be recognized by a constant heart rate of 80 to 90 beats/min at rest or during exercise. Patients with autonomic neuropathy are more likely to develop hypotension after vigorous exercise, particularly at the beginning of an exercise program (Vitug, Schneider, & Ruderman, 1988). They may have an elevated resting heart rate and reduced maximal heart rate. The rate of perceived exertion (RPE) may be the most appropriate measure for recommending exercise intensity because patients with neuropathy may exhibit chronotropic insufficiency during exercise. In addition, these individuals can have difficulty in thermoregulation and are prone to dehydration. Because they may also have a reduced ability to detect hypoglycemia, they require more careful glucose monitoring when initiating an exercise program. In addition, because there is a strong correlation between autonomic neuropathy and microvascular disease, similar exercise precautions should be taken.

Submaximal exercise testing is preferable if autonomic neuropathy is known to exist. A conservative approach to exercise testing in which inability to talk or maintain pedalling frequency are signals for termination is best. RPE is best used in prescribing exercise intensity because of hemodynamic abnormalities and the need to focus on the patient's subjective feelings. Water activities and stationary cycling are also recommended. If orthostatic (postural) hypotension is present, water exercise is particularly useful because the surrounding water pressure helps maintain blood pressure. Sitting exercises also maintain blood pressure.

Exercise Recommendations:

- Use submaximal testing (the test stops if the patient is unable to talk or maintain RPMs).
- Use RPE to gauge exercise intensity.
- Use water activities, stationary cycling or both (to maintain BP).

Exercise Precautions for Autonomic Neuropathy.   Avoid exercises that cause changes in body position and that are high-intensity; the risk of hypotension is too great, especially following strenuous exercise. Because patients with autonomic neuropathy have increased risk of dehydration and poor tolerance for the cold, they should avoid exercise in hot or cold environments. These patients should also be carefully monitored during and after exercise because they are prone to hypoglycemia. A summary of exercise precautions follows:

- Avoid high-intensity activity.
- Avoid rapid change in body position.
- Avoid extremes of temperature.
- Use careful glucose monitoring.

Peripheral Neuropathy

Peripheral neuropathies usually begin symmetrically in the lower and upper extremities (e.g., in the hands and feet) and progress proximally. The peripheral nerves have the ability to reenervate; therefore, widespread peripheral nerve damage is not clinically evident until the late stages. Neuropathy results in superficial or deep pain, impaired balance, numbness, loss of touch, and decreases in proprioception. It produces a deterioration of deep tendon reflexes, weakness in the hands and feet, and weakness and atrophy of the thigh muscles in some cases.

Exercise risks for people with peripheral neuropathy include these conditions:

- Superficial deep pain
- Impaired balance and reflexes
- Numbness and weakness in the hands and feet
- Decreased proprioception
- Weakness and atrophy of thigh muscles (when severe)

Exercise for Peripheral Neuropathy.   Activities that don't require weight bearing are suggested in the presence of neuropathy. Swimming, cycling, and arm exercises are suggested for those with insensitive feet to minimize trauma to the feet. Activities that improve awareness of the lower extremities and activities that teach balance are appropriate choices (Graham & Lasko-McCarthey, 1990). Patients with improved muscle function should be taught to stretch using props (e.g., towel or stick). RPE is very useful in determining the appropriate exercise intensity for these patients.

Problems associated with foot injury and peripheral circulation are important considerations for anyone with diabetes, but especially when the patient has a peripheral neuropathy. Close inspection of the feet and use of proper footwear should be emphasized, and the patient should avoid exercise that may cause trauma to the feet such as prolonged hiking, jogging, or walking on uneven surfaces. The patient should assess the feet regularly, taking careful note of blisters and calluses. Feet and toes should be kept clean and dry. Dry socks should always be used, and it is advisable to apply lotion regularly before bed and after bathing. It is especially important to choose a shoe that fits properly and has optimal cushioning (a number of shoes with special cushioning are available commercially). Stretching should be performed with caution—it should be done gently and should remain pain free. Signs of overstretching are muscle quivering and increasing pain as the stretch is held. Balance support such as chairs or railings may be necessary. Pulse monitoring may be inappropriate because of sensory loss in the fingers, another reason why RPE is preferable for these patients.

Exercise recommendations:

- Use RPE.
- Use nonweight-bearing activities (swimming, cycling, arm exercise).
- Use activities to improve balance.

Exercise Precautions for Peripheral Neuropathy.   Complications arising from peripheral neuropathies include ulceration of the feet and decreased healing ability. Severe *neuroarthropathy* can result in multiple fractures and dislocation of the bones of the feet and ankle without the patients' awareness. Although exercise cannot reverse the occurrence of peripheral neuropathy, it can be of benefit in preventing further loss of fitness associated with disuse. Range of motion activities for the major joints (i.e., ankle, knee, hip, trunk, shoulder, elbow, and wrist) should be performed to prevent or minimize contractures. A summary of exercise precautions follows:

- Take good care of the feet.
- Use proper footwear.
- Perform gentle, pain-free stretching.

Retinopathy

Some form of retinopathy is a common occurrence among those with diabetes. The incidence of diabetic retinopathy is directly proportional to the severity and duration of diabetes. Although the exact cause of diabetic retinopathy is unknown, recent findings suggest that intracellular sorbitol production by aldose reductase may contribute to diabetes-related pathology in many of the retinal cells. Retinopathy develops progressively. *Background retinopathy* is the early stage, and over time it may develop into *preproliferative retinopathy, proliferative retinopathy*, and eventually blindness. Retinopathy is aggravated by increases in intraocular pressure, and the pressure against weakened capillaries in the retina can cause rupture of the damaged vessels of the eye (Greenlee, 1987). Thus, exercise that increases blood pressure may worsen retinopathy. In addition, jarring the head during exercise (contact sports) could cause detachment of the retina. There is presently no clear evidence that intense exercise accelerates retinopathy. For these reasons, the effects of exercise on retinopathy warrant examination.

Sundkvist, Almar, Lilia, and Pandolfi (1984) evaluated growth hormone (GH) and endothelial function (factor VIII related antigen, VIII R:Ag and plasmogen activator activity, PAA) during exercise in 50 subjects with Type I diabetes. Factor VIII R:Ag measures the immunological activity of Von Willebrand factor, which promotes platelet adhesion and has been found to be elevated in patients with retinopathy (Pandolfi, Almar, & Holmberg, 1974). Twenty-four subjects (mean age 31 years) with diabetes of short to moderate duration (mean duration 11 years) and 26 subjects (mean age 55 years) with long-duration (mean duration 35 years) diabetes were studied. Half the patients in each group had signs of retinopathy. The subjects with short duration of diabetes who showed a significant increase in growth hormone during exercise were those with signs of retinopathy. Among those with diabetes of short duration, VIII R:Ag and PAA increased earlier and more markedly in subjects with retinopathy. In patients with diabetes of long duration there were no differences in GH, VIII R:Ag or PAA between those with and without retinopathy. In patients with diabetes of short duration, these findings indicate metabolic differences in response to exercise between those with and those without retinopathy. These findings, however, have not been extended clinically; further research is needed to confirm results and clarify their clinical significance.

Exercise Risks:

- Elevations in blood pressure
- Jarring of the head (possible retinal detachment)

Exercise for Diabetic Retinopathy.   For the individual with proliferative retinopathy, a *submaximal exercise test* should be conducted to establish a training heart rate, or rate of perceived exertion, based on blood pressure response. A systolic blood pressure response of 200 mmHg or above risks further damage to the retina. Greenlee (1987) recommended that heart rates not exceed the rate that elicits a systolic BP (SBP) of 170 mmHg for individuals with proliferative retinopathy. If proliferative retinopathy is present, patients should exercise at a facility where BP response can be monitored. If this is not possible, patients should be monitored initially, and their heart rates and RPEs should be used to design outpatient programs.

Exercise resulting in large increases in systolic pressure (i.e., *Valsalva maneuvers* such as heavy weight lifting, stretching with breath holding, bending, or head stands, as well as high-intensity aerobic activity) can cause retinal hemorrhage if proliferative retinopathy is present. Aerobic exercise for these patients could include stationary cycling, walking, swimming, and low-intensity rowing on a rowing machine.

Exercise Recommendations:

- Use HR and RPE based on BP response.
- Maintain SBP below 170 mmHg during exercise.
- Use low-impact activities.

Exercise Recommendations for Proliferative Retinopathy:

- Use a submaximal exercise test (use HR or RPE based on BP response).
- Maintain SBP below 170 mmHg during exercise.
- Use stationary cycling, walking, swimming, or low-intensity rowing.
- If possible, monitor BP during exercise.

Exercise Precautions for Diabetic Retinopathy.   In patients with background retinopathy, exercise does not have to be monitored as closely as with proliferative retinopathy, but activities that do not increase blood pressure excessively (greater than 180 mmHg) and are low impact are most suitable. Caution should be taken when performing strenuous upper extremity exercise (e.g., arm cycle ergometer) because the increase in peripheral resistance to blood flow increases blood pressure. If the patient has recently undergone retinal photocoagulation treatment or eye surgery, exercise is contraindicated. A summary of exercise precautions follows:

- Avoid Valsalva maneuvers.
- Avoid heavy weight lifting, breath-holding stretches, high-intensity exercise, and strenuous upper arm exercise.
- Exercise is contraindicated if the individual has had recent photocoagulation treatment or surgery.

Nephropathy

As many as 48% of patients diagnosed with diabetes before age 20 die from renal insufficiency an average of 22 years after the onset of diabetes (Balodimos, 1971). Early detection of renal damage might allow selective management to offset disease progression. Exercise has been suggested as a possible means of assessing nephropathy.

Mogensen and Vittinghus (1975) proposed an exercise stress test as a means of screening for the early presence of albuminuria in diabetic adults. Several studies have determined the utility of exercise as a means of identifying those at increased risk of developing nephropathy. Although data are conflicting, it appears that exercise can lead to increased urinary albumin excretion in a large number of patients (Poortmans, Dorchy, & Toussiant, 1982). Research in this area has shown only a weak correlation or no correlation between systemic hemodynamics during exercise and albumin excretion (Huttunen, Kaar, Pietilainen, Vierikko, & Reinila, 1981; Torffit, Castenfors, Bengtsson, & Agardh, 1987). Due to the limitations in sensitivity and specificity of this finding, the use of exercise to screen patients for nephropathy is not widely practiced. These results indicate the potential prognostic information of exercise testing. However, the actual use of exercise testing in determining the long-term outcome for these patients has not been documented.

Ala-Houhala (1990) found that when comparing healthy controls to patients with insulin-dependent diabetes who exhibit mild *proteinuria*, exercise resulted in a significant reduction in glomerular filtration rate (GFR) and renal plasma flow (RPF) in both groups. The reduction in GFR was small compared with the decrease in RPF, as has been previously shown (Poortmans, 1985; Vittinghus & Mogensen, 1981). Thus the filtration fraction (FF) markedly increased in both patients and controls. The fractional clearance of albumin was significantly increased in both groups, whereas fractional clearance of IgG increased significantly only in the patients. The patient group had a significant elevation in the fractional clearance of molecules with a radius of greater than or equal to 4.8 nm after exercise, which was not found in controls. Correlational analysis revealed the possibility that the exercise-induced rise in fractional protein clearance could be a consequence of an increase in FF. Like Vittinghaus and Mogensen (1981), Ala-Houhala (1990) found no significant relationship between changes in systolic blood pressure and protein clearance.

These researchers concluded that exercise increases the permeability of the glomeruli by greatly influencing the renal hemodynamics, shown by the increase in FF. Depletion of negative charges on the glomerular capillary wall at least partially influences the exercise-induced proteinuria in both healthy controls and patients with insulin-dependent diabetes. In addition, the alteration in glomerular permeability during exercise is associated with an increase in the filtering pores in patients with diabetic nephropathy. These findings add information about the mechanisms behind the changes in protein clearance that occur with exercise and the differences between patients and controls. The influence of exercise on the clinical status of patients with nephropathy warrants further investigation.

Almost all the known risk factors for CVD are more prevalent in renal patients undergoing dialysis, including elevated serum cholesterol, triglyceride and LDL cholesterol levels, decreased HDL cholesterol levels, hypertension, elevated fibrinogen, glucose intolerance, hyperinsulinemia, and a sedentary lifestyle. A role for exercise is indicated by these risk factors in patients. An exercise program must be carefully developed based on the patient's degree of kidney damage. An excellent source of information on exercise for the patient in end-stage renal disease (ESRD) who is undergoing dialysis is the work of Painter (Painter, 1988). Exercise training for patients undergoing dialysis has been shown to bring about improvements in serum lipids, blood pressure, and maximal oxygen consumption (Goldberg, Hagberg, Delmez, Florman, & Harter, 1979; Painter & Zimmerman, 1986).

Exercise Risks:

- Marked changes in hemodynamics
- Marked elevations in BP
- Presence of retinopathy likely

Exercise for Nephropathy.   In general, vigorous exercise that results in marked changes in hemodynamics should be avoided in patients with renal problems. This could include lifting heavy weights and high-intensity aerobic activities. Because many patients who have clinical diabetic nephropathy often have elevated blood pressure at rest, marked increases in blood pressure should be avoided, for example, any activity that requires breath holding or the Valsalva maneuver.

The most preferable activities for people with nephropathy are dynamic. However, some precautions need to be taken not only with regard to intensity, but also with the effects of impact. Renal osteodystrophy is a common occurrence among patients with nephropathy and begins early when renal function begins to decline; therefore, dynamic activities that are weight bearing, yet low impact, are preferable. In addition, shoes with some type of cushioning system (e.g., gel or air) are recommended. Submaximal isometric or light weight lifting may be appropriate to maintain muscle tone, as long as blood pressure is controlled and left ventricular function is normal. Because the microvascular diseases are correlated with the presence of nephropathy, retinopathy may also be likely, so these individuals need to be cautious in activities that elevate BP. As previously mentioned, specific training programs for patients undergoing hemodialysis are advised (Painter, 1988).

Exercise Recommendations:

- Include dynamic, weight-bearing, low-impact activities.
- Use submaximal isometric or light weight lifting when BP is controlled and left ventricular function is normal.
- Develop specific programs for hemodialysis patients (See Painter).

Exercise Precautions for Nephropathy. Renal patients need to be fully evaluated before beginning to exercise. Nephropathy is a multisystem disease, and all systems need to be assessed carefully. An exercise program should not begin until the patient has been stabilized on medication, dialysis when indicated, and diet. Fluid replacement is extremely important in these patients because of the effects of fluid balance changes on blood pressure. It is unclear if exercise accelerates nephropathy; however, because sustained elevations in blood pressure do accelerate diabetic nephropathy, it would seem prudent to avoid activities involving sustained blood pressure elevation (Vitug et al., 1988).

Thus the importance of careful screening for underlying complications is evident. Complications require special consideration and precautions. A summary of exercise precautions follows:

- Avoid lifting weights, intense aerobic activities and Valsalva maneuvers.
- Use cushioned shoes (e.g., gel, air).
- Maintain hydration.

Follow-Up

In the early stages of an exercise program, the patient should be reexamined every 3 to 6 months to evaluate adaptation, adherence, and possible benefits of the exercise program. Glycemic control (HbA$_1$) should be evaluated. When it is possible for the patient to arrive fasting, a lipid profile should be obtained (total cholesterol, triglycerides, HDL cholesterol, LDL cholesterol) if initial abnormalities in blood lipids were noted. Height, weight, and insulin dose should be recorded, and the patient should be asked to fill out a simple questionnaire on dietary intake, physical activity patterns, regular blood glucose monitoring, and hypoglycemic occurrences over the past month. Exercise prescriptions should be evaluated and, if necessary, updated. For patients who are successful with their exercise programs and who do not need close monitoring or special supervision, further reading is recommended (see *Diabetes: Your Complete Guide to Exercise* by Neil Gordon, Human Kinetics: Champaign, IL, 1993).

Some potentially fruitful areas of future clinical research include

- long-term follow-up (CVD risk),
- exercise for transplant patients, and
- specific exercise recommendations (type and intensity)

Case Studies

The following are typical case studies of patients receiving exercise therapy.

■■■■■ CASE STUDY 1

A 35-year-old, 5 ft 4 in., 135 lb female with Type I diabetes is found after initial examination to have background retinopathy, some peripheral neuropathy, resting blood pressure of 130/80, pulse of 80 bts/min, and a hemoglobin A_1 of 11%. She wants to begin an aerobics class that meets two to three times a week to lose 10 to 15 lb.

A low-impact aerobics class is recommended. The importance of a low-impact class is emphasized because of the risk high-impact aerobics would carry of bone stress and aggravating the existing retinopathy. Because of the partial neuropathy the importance of shoes with a proper fit, good support, and cushioning should be emphasized. The patient should check her feet after each exercise session for blisters or abrasions to the feet that could otherwise go unnoticed.

Based on the results of a graded exercise test (GXT), a target heart rate (THR) and rating of perceived exertion (RPE) for exercise were given. In this case the recommendations were a THR of 133 to 140 bts/ min, representing 50% to 60% of maximum capacity at a point prior to the anaerobic threshold. This level was equivalent to an RPE of 14. The individual was taken through several aerobics sessions during which her heart rate was monitored, and she learned to monitor her own RPE. After this, spot-checking of pulse during exercise was recommended.

Because of her interest in being active and losing weight, a lower to moderate level of activity was recommended. If the program is well tolerated, the level can be increased to 60% to 70% (140 to 150 bts/min THR) after 3 months. Initially blood glucose should be checked before, immediately after, and 15 min to 1 hr after each exercise session to determine her particular response to exercise, including possible hypoglycemia, and to assess whether the intensity of exercise may be too high (hyperglycemia).

This individual is on a mixed split-dose insulin regimen consisting of 20 units of Lente and 10 units of regular insulin in the morning and evening. Because the aerobics class is at 8:00 a.m., it is recommended that she reduce the morning short-acting insulin by 50% (5 units) or eliminate it altogether, depending on her blood glucose response to exercise. She was advised to check blood glucose before the noon meal and evening insulin dose to evaluate if the evening dose needs adjusting. Careful glucose monitoring should be initiated and continued for the first 6 weeks of the program. Reductions in insulin are the main response advised because weight loss is desired; however, should frequent hypoglycemia occur, supplemental caloric intake may be required.

The subject will return in 6 weeks for evaluation of her progress in the program. Weight loss should be checked and records of blood glucose and occurrence of hypoglycemia should also be discussed at this time. After 12 weeks the hemoglobin A_1 should be rechecked and weight loss and target heart rate reevaluated. If the program is tolerated well and progress is being achieved, an increase in the training load to 60% to 70% of maximum capacity (140 to 150 THR) can be recommended. After the target weight (120 lbs) is achieved, recommendations for supplemental food can be given in conjunction with continued exercise to maintain weight.

Example Exercise Program for Case 1

The patient chose low-impact aerobics and walking as an alternative exercise. Her program included low-impact aerobics 2 to 3 days per week with walking on alternate days for 3 to 5 days a week of exercise.

Warm-up.   10 min of stretching and flexibility exercises done seated without head lowering (because of the presence of some retinopathy).

Stimulus.   5 min at an easy pace to gradually increase heart rate.

20 to 25 min to gradually increase the heart rate to the THR (walking 15 min per mile).

5 min to cool down at an easy pace to decrease the heart rate.

Cool down.   5 to 10 min of stretching and abdominal exercises (curl-ups with bent knees and feet anchored that require slightly raising shoulders off the ground). Use light (5 lb) hand weights for biceps curls and shoulder shrugs.

Comments.   Most stretching and flexibility exercises can be used; however, this patient should avoid exercises that lower the head or require bouncing or holding the breath because of background retinopathy. She should check her feet regularly because of her peripheral neuropathy. The aerobics class should be low impact, incorporating stretching, strength training (using light hand weights), and cardiovascular endurance with no jumping. Blood glucose should be checked before and after exercise to determine if modifications in insulin dose are necessary.

■■■■   **CASE STUDY 2**

A 45-year-old, 5 ft 11 in., 170 lb male with Type I diabetes since age 16 was found upon screening to have proliferative retinopathy and autonomic neuropathy, mild hypertension (140/90), pulse 76, and hemoglobin A_1 of 9%. This man would like to exercise to lower his blood pressure and to become more active because he has an office job and gets minimal daily activity. Based on his initial screening, a low-impact, low-intensity program (because of his existing retinopathy) is recommended. A GXT is required and recommendations are given. Submaximal testing should be used because proliferative retinopathy is present, and exercise intensity should be established based on blood pressure response.

Because autonomic neuropathy can affect heart rate, guidelines for training based on blood pressure response and RPE are given. An RPE of 12 to 13 is recommended as a training level because a systolic blood pressure response of 170 was reached at an RPE of 14. The specific modes of exercise chosen were cycling and swimming because these activities are minimal impact, can be low intensity, and do not cause marked increases in blood pressure. An initial program of four to five exercise sessions per week, alternating cycling and swimming, is advised. The patient comes to the clinic two times for cycling sessions in which blood glucose, blood pressure, and RPE are monitored. Since this individual has proliferative retinopathy, he is given an in-house program in which his blood pressure can be monitored during exercise sessions.

Insulin treatment consists of a single dose of 30 units of Lente and 20 NPH. Minor adjustments in insulin (primarily reductions in NPH) were recommended based on glucose monitoring. Advice on supplemental carbohydrate use was given. Follow-up sessions at 6 weeks and 12 weeks were scheduled with the diabetes management team. At follow-up, proliferative retinopathy, resting BP, and glucose records should be evaluated. In addition, hemoglobin A_1 should be checked at the 12-week follow-up meeting.

Example Exercise Program for Case 2

The patient chose cycling and swimming for the exercise program. Exercise should take place 3 to 5 days a week.

Warm-up.   5 min at an easy pace (cycling 15 to 20 mph with slight resistance). 5 min of stretching, seated without bouncing or breath holding.

Stimulus.   Swimming or cycling.

20 to 25 min to increase an RPE of 12 to 13 (systolic blood pressure monitored less than 170 mmHg).

5 min at an easy pace to gradually lower the intensity of exercise.

Cool down.   5 to 10 min of stretching, use of some light hand weights (5-10 lb) for upper body strengthening.

Comments. Monitor blood pressure during cycling sessions. Avoid heavy weight lifting because of hypertension and proliferative retinopathy. RPE should be used for exercise sessions because of the presence of autonomic neuropathy. Swimming laps is also recommended as an alternative exercise to cycling and can be used on alternate days. Blood glucose should be checked before and after exercise to determine if alterations in insulin dose, dietary intake, or both are necessary.

References

Ala-Houhala, I. (1990). Effects of exercise on glomerular passage of macromolecules in patients with diabetic nephropathy and in healthy subjects. *Scandinavian Journal of Clinical and Laboratory Investigation,* **50,** 27-33.

Balodimos, N.C. (1971). Diabetic nephropathy. In A. Marble (Ed.), *Joslin's diabetes mellitus* (p. 526). Philadelphia: Lea and Febiger.

Berger, M., Halban, P.A., Assal, J.P., Offord, R.E., Vranic, M., & Renold, A.E. (1979). Pharmokinetics of subcutaneously injected tritiated insulin: Effects of exercise. *Diabetes,* **28**(Suppl. I), 53-57.

Bergstrom, B., Manhem, P., Bramnert, M., Lilia, B., & Sundkvist, G. (1989). Impaired responses of catecholamines to exercise in diabetic patients with abnormal heart rate reactions to tilt. *Clinical Physiology,* **9,** 259-267.

Bernbaum, M., Albert, S.G., & Cohen, J.D. (1989). Exercise training in individuals with diabetic retinopathy and blindness. *Archives of Physical Medicine and Rehabilitation,* **70,** 605-611.

Binder, C., Lauritzen, T., Faber, O., & Pramming, S. (1984). Insulin pharmacokinetics. *Diabetes Care,* **7,** 188-199.

Campaigne, B.N. (1988). Evaluation and testing of the diabetic patient prior to exercise prescription. In L.K. Hall & G.C. Meyer (Eds.), *Epidemiology behavior change and intervention in chronic disease* (pp. 167-177). Champaign, IL: LaCrosse Exercise and Health Series, Life Enhancement Publications.

Coyle, E.F., & Coyle, E. (1993). Carbohydrates that speed recovery from training. *Physician and Sports Medicine,* **21,** 111-123.

Ewing, D.J., Bellavere, F., Espi, F., McKibben, R.M., Buchanan, K.D., Biemersma, P.A., & Clarke, B.F. (1986). Correlation of cardiovascular and neuroendocrine tests of autonomic function in diabetes. *Metabolism,* **35,** 349-353.

Ewing, D.J., Campbell, L.W., & Clarke, B.F. (1981). Heart rate changes in diabetes mellitus. *Lancet,* **1,** 183-186.

Ewing, D.J., & Clark, B.J. (1982). Diagnosis and management of diabetic autonomic neuropathy. *British Medical Journal,* **285,** 916-918.

Ewing, D.J., Martyn, C.N., Young, R.J., & Clarke, B.F. (1985). The value of cardiovascular autonomic function tests: Ten years experience in diabetes. *Diabetes Care, 8,* 491-498.

Federlin, K., Laube, H., & Velcovsky, H.G. (1981). Biologic and immunologic in vivo and in vitro studies with biosynthetic human insulin. *Diabetes Care, 4,* 170-174.

Fernqvist, E., Linde, B., Ostman, J., & Gunnarsson, R. (1986). Effects of physical exercise on insulin absorption in insulin-dependent diabetics. A comparison between human and porcine insulin. *Clinical Physiology, 6,* 489-498.

Frid, A., & Linde, B. (1986). Where do lean diabetics inject their insulin? A study using computed tomography. *British Medical Journal, 292,* 1638.

Frid, A., Ostman, J., & Linde, B. (1990). Hypoglycemia risk during and after intramuscular injection of insulin in thigh in IDDM. *Diabetes Care, 13,* 473-477.

Goldberg, A.P., Hagberg, J.M., Delmez, J.A., Florman, F.W., & Harter, H.R. (1979). Exercise training improves abnormal lipid and carbohydrate metabolism in hemodialysis patients. *Transamerican Society of Artificial Internal Organs, 25,* 431-436.

Graham, C., & Lasko-McCarthey, P. (1990). Exercise options for persons with diabetic complications. *Diabetes Educator, 16,* 212-220.

Greenlee, G. (1987). Exercise options for patients with retinopathy and peripheral vascular disease. *Practical Diabetology, 6*(4), 9-11.

Haffner, S.M., Stern, M.P., Mazuda, H.P., Mitchell, B.D., & Patterson, J.K. (1990). Cardiovascular risk factors in confirmed prediabetic individuals: Does the clock for coronary heart disease start ticking before the onset of clinical diabetes? *Journal of the American Medical Association, 263*(21), 2893-2898.

Hilsted, J., Galbo, H., & Christensen, N.J. (1979). Impaired cardiovascular responses to graded exercise in diabetic autonomic neuropathy. *Diabetes, 28*(4), 313-319.

Hilsted, J., Galbo, H., & Christensen, N.J. (1980). Impaired responses of catecholamines, growth hormone and cortisol to graded exercise in diabetic autonomic neuropathy. *Diabetes, 29*(4), 257-262.

Hilsted, J., Galbo, H., Christensen, N.J., Parving, H.H., & Benn, J. (1982). Haemodynamic changes during graded exercise in patients with diabetic autonomic neuropathy. *Diabetologia, 22,* 318-323.

Hoeldtke, R.D., Boden, G., Shuman, C.R., & Owen, O.E. (1982). Reduced epinephrine secretion and hypoglycemia unawareness in diabetic autonomic neuropathy. *Annals of Internal Medicine, 96,* 459-462.

Hoeldtke, R.D., & Cilmi, K.M., (1984). Norepinephrine secretion and production in diabetic autonomic neuropathy. *Journal of Clinical Endocrinology and Metabolism, 59,* 246-252.

Horton, E.S. (1988). Role and management of exercise in diabetes mellitus. *Diabetes Care, 11*(2), 201-211.

Huttunen, N.P., Kaar, M.L., Pietilainen, M., Vierikko, P., & Reinila, M. (1981). Exercise-induced proteinuria in children and adolescents. *Scandinavian Journal of Clinical and Laboratory Investigation*, **41**, 583-587.

Kahn, J.K., Zola, B., Juni, I.E., & Vinik, A.I. (1986). Decreased exercise heart rate and blood pressure response in diabetic subjects with cardiac autonomic neuropathy. *Diabetes Care*, **9**(4), 389-394.

Karlefors, T. (1966). Exercise tests in male diabetics. *Acta Medica Scandinavica*, **180**(Suppl. 449), 3-80.

Koivisto, V.A., & Felig, P. (1978). Effects of leg exercise on insulin absorption in diabetic patients. *New England Journal of Medicine*, **298**, 79-83.

Koivisto, V.A., & Felig, P. (1980). Alterations in insulin absorption and in blood glucose control associated with varying insulin injection sites in diabetic patients. *Annals of Internal Medicine*, **92**, 59-61.

Margonato, A., Grundini, P., Vicedomini, G., Gilardi, M.C., Pozza, G., & Fazio, F. (1986). Abnormal cardiovascular response to exercise in young asymptomatic diabetic patients with retinopathy. *American Heart Journal*, **112**(3), 554-560.

Martin, M.J., Robbins, D.C., Bergenstal, R., LaGrange, B., & Rubenstein, A.H. (1982). Absence of exercise-induced hypoglycemia in Type I (insulin-dependent) diabetic patients during maintenance of normoglycemia, by short-term, open-loop insulin infusion. *Diabetologia*, **23**, 337-342.

Mogensen, C.E., & Vittinghus, K. (1975). Urinary albumin excretion during exercise in juvenile diabetes. A provocation test for early abnormalities. *Scandinavian Journal of Clinical and Laboratory Investigation*, **32**, 295-300.

Painter, P. (1988). Exercise in end-stage renal disease. *Exercise and Sports Science Reviews*, **16**, 305-340.

Painter, P., & Zimmerman, S. (1986). Exercise in end-stage renal disease. *American Journal of Kidney Diseases*, **7**, 386-394.

Pandolfi, M., Almar, L.O., & Holmberg, L. (1974). Increased vonWillebrand-antihaemophilic factor A in diabetic retinopathy. *Acta Ophthalmologica*, **52**, 823-828.

Poortmans, J.R. (1985). Postexercise proteinuria in humans: Facts and mechanisms. *Journal of the American Medical Association*, **253**, 236-240.

Poortmans, J., Dorchy, H., & Toussiant, D. (1982). Urinary excretion of total proteins, albumin and beta 2-microalbumin during rest and exercise in diabetic adolescents with and without retinopathy. *Diabetes Care*, **5**(6), 617-623.

Pramming, S., Lauritzen, T., Thorsteinsson, B., Johansen, K., & Binder, C. (1984). Absorption of soluble and isophane semisynthetic human and porcine insulin in insulin-dependent subjects. *Acta Endocrinologica*, **105**, 215-220.

Ruegemer, J., Squires, R.W., Marsh, H.M., Haymond, M.W., Cryer, P.E., Rizza, R.A., & Miles, J.M. (1990). Differences between prebreakfast and late afternoon glycemic response to exercise in IDDM patients. *Diabetes Care,* **13**, 104-110.

Schiffrin, A., Parikh, S., Marliss, E.B., & Desrosiers, M.M. (1984). Metabolic response to fasting exercise in adolescent insulin-dependent diabetic subjects treated with continuous subcutaneous insulin infusion and intensive conventional therapy. *Diabetes Care,* **7**, 255-260.

Sonnenberg, G.E., Kemmer, F.W., & Berger, M. (1990). Exercise in Type I (insulin dependent) diabetic patients treated with continuous subcutaneous insulin infusion. Prevention of exercise induced hypoglycemia. *Diabetologia,* **33**, 696-703.

Stout, R.W. (1979). Diabetes and atherosclerosis—The role of insulin. *Diabetologia,* **16**, 141-150.

Sundkvist, G., Almar, A.O., Lilia, B., & Pandolfi, M. (1984). Growth hormone and endothelial function during exercise in diabetics with and without retinopathy. *Acta Medica Scandinavica,* **215**, 55-61.

Torffit, O., Castenfors, J., Bengtsson, U., & Agardh, C.D. (1987). Exercise stimulation in insulin-dependent diabetics, normal increase in albuminuria with abnormal blood pressure response. *Scandinavian Journal of Clinical and Laboratory Investigation,* **47**, 253-259.

Valbona, C. (1982). Bodily responses to immobilization. In F.J. Kottke, G.K. Stillwell, & J.F. Lehman (Eds.), *Kruzen Handbook of Physical Medicine and Rehabilitation* (3rd ed.) (pp. 963-975). Philadelphia: W.B. Saunders.

Vittinghus, E., & Mogensen, C.E. (1981). Albumin excretion and renal hemodynamic response to physical exercise in normal and diabetic man. *Scandinavian Journal of Clinical and Laboratory Investigation,* **4**, 627-632.

Vitug, A., Schneider, S.H., & Ruderman, N.B. (1988). Exercise and type I diabetes mellitus. In K.B. Pandolf (Ed.), *Exercise and Sports Sciences Reviews,* **16** (pp. 285-304). New York: MacMillan.

Zinman, B., Murray, F.T., Vranic, M., Albisser, A.M., Leibel, B.S., McClean, P.A., & Marliss, E.B. (1977). Glucosegulation during moderate exercise in insulin treated diabetics. *Journal of Clinical Endocrinology and Metabolism,* **45**, 641-652.

Zinman, B., Vranic, M., Albisser, A.M., Leibel, B.S., & Marliss, E.B. (1979). The role of insulin in metabolic response to exercise in diabetic man. *Diabetes,* **28**, 76-81.

Chapter

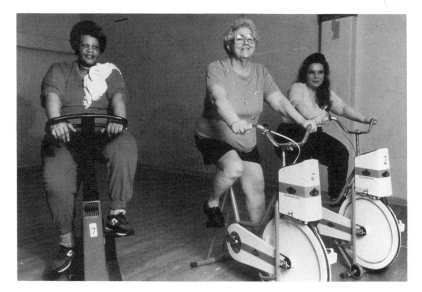

The Clinical Application of Exercise in Type II Diabetes

We have documented well in earlier chapters the known physical and metabolic benefits of exercise training for the person with Type II diabetes. But the suitability of exercise training is still often questioned in those with circulatory and other medical problems. All patients should have their underlying medical problems thoroughly evaluated to be sure that exercise training can be effectively and safely performed. The number and severity of complications that may be present usually relate to how long the diabetes has existed. Severe complications include cardiovascular, neurological, and end-stage organ disease. Common complications associated with Type II diabetes are

- silent ischemia,
- hypertension,
- retinopathy,
- sensory and autonomic neuropathy,

- nephropathy,
- peripheral vascular disease, and
- proteinuria.

If begun early in life, exercise training may help to normalize many of these pathologies and may even prevent them. People at high risk for developing NIDDM may benefit from exercise because it may delay the onset of the disease. Individuals with overt Type II diabetes can also benefit psychologically, as shown in Table 7.1.

More short-term and long-term, primary prevention, secondary prevention, and tertiary trials of the efficacy of exercise training as a therapeutic intervention are still needed to more fully delineate the role of physical training (King & Kriska, 1992). Present knowledge suggests that to be most effective, individualized exercise prescriptions should be provided alone or in combination with dietary modifications or drug therapy (or both) to optimize treatment for Type II diabetes. Younger, nonobese people with a family history of Type II diabetes are likely to benefit from a relatively high-intensity exercise program. People who are middle-aged or older, obese, and have mild to moderate glucose intolerance and insulin resistance should undergo moderate-intensity exercise therapy in combination with dietary intervention. Those who are older, obese, and have more severe complications of diabetes may also use low-intensity exercise training together with diet or drug therapy as part of their overall therapeutic management.

There are potential risks to exercise and it may be contraindicated for some patients with diabetes, but these risks can be minimized if patients have a good knowledge of their medical and physical limitations, of their physiological response to exercise, and of how to exercise appropriately. With this knowledge, they can exercise safely and enjoy the benefits of this effective intervention modality. The person with diabetes is not at a markedly greater risk for exercise-induced complications when appropriate precautions are taken. An individualized exercise program based

Table 7.1 Potential Changes in Psychological Parameters With Exercise Training

Measure	Change
Depression	Decreases
Self-esteem	Increases
General feeling of well-being	Increases
Positive attitude toward work	Increases
Self-confidence	Increases

on sound medical and physiological principles can account for most limitations and allow the person with Type II diabetes to enjoy a safe and effective dynamic exercise program. It is important to note that not only does exercise training provide effective therapy, but it provides people with diabetes an opportunity to lead more normal and active lifestyles.

Before embarking on a vigorous physical exercise program, anyone with diabetes should undergo complete medical, physical, and laboratory testing and discuss with his or her physician the potential effect of exercise on any required medications. Any patient with NIDDM should probably undergo an exercise stress test, especially if cardiac disease exists or is suspected. Recommendations and guidelines for prescribing exercise should be individualized and take into account diet and insulin or oral hypoglycemic agents. Extra precautions often need consideration when prescribing exercise training for those not engaged in a supervised program. It is best to thoroughly explain potential complications that may affect compliance with an exercise program to each individual before he or she embarks on it. Recommendations that should be systematically followed to ensure the successful management and safety of patients with NIDDM undergoing exercise therapy follow.

Screening and Medical Evaluation

The presence of central and android obesity (Bergstrom et al., 1990; Ohlson et al., 1985) should be useful in identifying patients with a high likelihood of developing NIDDM or patients who are diabetic but unaware that they have this disease. An oral glucose tolerance test is useful in both assessing the degree of glucose impairment and characterizing insulin secretion patterns. Insulin resistance and hyperinsulinemia are events known to precede the clinical onset of Type II diabetes (Lillioja & Bogardus, 1988; Warren, Martin, Krolewski, Soeldner, & Kahn, 1990). A simple approach for screening individuals for the possibility of insulin resistance is to measure for elevated fasting glucose levels. Direct methods to measure in vivo insulin resistance (the euglycemic clamp test) are complicated and are beyond the capabilities of most clinical approaches.

Individuals who have had Type II diabetes for over 30 years are at high risk for underlying coronary artery disease (Reaven, 1988). If a patient shows symptoms of coronary artery disease, a complete cardiology evaluation, including an exercise stress test, should be performed. Stress test results should be evaluated for a number of conditions, especially those associated with accelerated atherosclerosis. An example for standard screening of patients was given in chapter 6 (see Table 6.1). Coronary artery disease, peripheral vascular occlusive arterial disease, and stroke are the major causes for morbidity and mortality in those with NIDDM (Ruderman & Haudenschild, 1984). Once proper evaluation is made and any previously undiagnosed problem is medically treated, the benefits of exercise as a therapeutic modality usually outweigh the risks.

Potential Adverse Effects of Physical Training

Although exercise is often recommended for patients with Type II diabetes, potentially adverse effects may occur with exercise, as shown in Table 7.2.

These potential complications can be minimized by developing an individualized exercise program. The clinical management team and information from its members' areas of specialization (i.e., endocrinology, exercise physiology, nutrition, and diabetes education) are important to optimize the patient's management, safety, compliance, and success. The major task of the team involves the long-term motivation of middle-aged individuals who are usually sedentary to develop physically active lifestyles. Boredom and lack of time, rather than medical problems, are the usual reason patients give for poor compliance with an exercise program.

Table 7.2   Potential Adverse Effects of Exercise in Type II Diabetes

Parameter	Adverse effects
Metabolic	• Hyperglycemia/ketosis (insulin therapy) • Hypoglycemia (insulin/sulfonylurea therapy)
Cardiovascular	• Ischemic heart disease and related cardiac dysfunction and arrhythmias leading to inadequate cardiac function, myocardial infarction, or both • Abnormal blood pressure response • Abnormal chronotropic response • Severe extremity claudication associated with advanced peripheral vascular occlusive arterial disease
Microvascular	• Proteinuria • Advanced microvascular lesions • Retinal hemorrhage
Musculoskeletal	• Degenerative joint disease • Orthopedic injuries • Foot ulcerations related to neuropathy

From "Clinical Practice Recommendations" by the American Diabetes Association, 1990-1991, *Diabetes Care*, **14**(Suppl. 2), p. 53. Copyright 1991 by American Diabetes Association, Inc. Adapted by permission.

Preexercise Training Evaluation

Before an individualized exercise program is recommended, a patient should undergo a physical examination. A graded exercise test is ideal for everyone and is necessary if clinically indicated (American College of Sports Medicine Guidelines for Graded Exercise Testing, 1991). A patient over the age of 35 with known risk factors for coronary artery disease should also undergo an exercise stress test including a multilead electrocardiogram for evaluation of

- silent ischemia,
- a marked hypertensive response to exercise, and
- abnormal orthostatic response following exercise.

The results of the exercise stress test are useful in formulating an individualized exercise prescription, and the test can be an effective means for showing patients that they can exercise safely.

Exercise Prescription: Systematic Approach

Relatively healthy younger individuals with mild NIDDM usually can follow an individualized exercise program as recommended for the general population (American College of Sports Medicine Guidelines for Exercise Testing and Prescription, 1991). These guidelines can easily be modified to account for a patient's limitations. Because its benefits have a limited duration, exercise must be performed routinely, at least every second day. Table 7.3 shows exercise recommendations and guidelines. Cardiorespiratory, muscular strength, and psychological changes are specific to training techniques and depend on the mode of activity, intensity

Table 7.3   Exercise Recommendations for Relatively Healthy NIDDM

Component	Recommendation
Type	Aerobic: walking, jogging, cycling, stair climbing, cross country ski machine, etc. Strength training (moderate level resistance training): circuit programs using light weights with 10-15 reps
Intensity	70%-85% maximum heart rate or 50%-70% $\dot{V}O_2$max
Duration	20-60 min plus a 5-10 min warm-up and cool-down period
Frequency	3-5 times weekly; daily if on insulin therapy.

of effort, duration of activity, and frequency of exercise. These components should be integrated into a well-constructed, systematic program for total fitness. Exercise training should always begin at a low-intensity level and progress slowly with respect to intensity and duration of effort.

Modes of Activity

Activities that are rhythmic, dynamic, and that use large muscle groups enhance cardiovascular fitness, weight control, and muscular strength. Such activities include walking, jogging, swimming, aerobic dancing, biking, rowing, and the like. These are referred to as aerobic exercises because they require an adequate oxygen supply to the contracting muscles to sustain the activity. For the individual with NIDDM, it is important that these exercises do not traumatize the feet, especially in those with peripheral vascular occlusive arterial disease, peripheral neuropathy, or both.

Muscular activities involving resistance exercises using exercise machines or light weights and involving a high number of repetitions result in muscular tone, strength, and endurance. Contrary to earlier concerns, a program of light resistance training can be safe and effective if performed properly (Durak, Jovanovic-Peterson, & Peterson, 1990; Goldberg, 1989; Miller, Sherman, & Ivy, 1984; Yki-Järvinen & Koivisto, 1983). In performing these activities, it is important that patients do not perform the Valsalva maneuver, which could result in a marked increase in systolic blood pressure. It has been recommended that systolic blood pressure remain under 180 mmHg during exercise (Bernbaum, Albert, Cohen, & Drimmer, 1989).

It is important that the patient enjoys the activities chosen and that they fit into her or his lifestyle. Incorporating many activities in the patient's program provides variety and usually reduces the boredom associated with exercise training. Including family members is important, so some activities should be those that the patient can do with them. This is one reason why walking is an excellent way to exercise. The patient can perform the exercise activity chosen in a formal setting or alone. These considerations about the mode of activity should effectively help promote adherence and compliance and combat recidivism.

Warm-Up and Cool-Down Periods

Low-intensity aerobic exercise performed for 5 to 10 min should be used to warm up and cool down. The warm-up prepares the body for more strenuous exercise. The cool-down period allows the body to gradually return to a resting state. Slow walking is an excellent way to cool down. Static stretching (sustained muscle stretching lasting 10 to 15 sec or longer) helps maintain flexibility and joint range of motion and may help prevent injuries when performed before, and especially following, exercise. The stretch should be held firm to the point where a comfortable pull is felt on the muscle for approximately 15 sec. The static stretch should be repeated four times for each muscle group. The person can take a short rest of 10 sec between stretches. A regular breathing pattern should be maintained while stretching to prevent a Valsalva response.

Intensity of Effort

A patient should start an exercise program with a low intensity of effort and progress slowly as she or he becomes stronger. The intensity of exercise, as monitored by an exercise-induced heart rate (HR) response (exercise training HR or $HR_{exer\,tr}$), can be prescribed as a percentage of the patient's heart rate at maximal effort (HR_{max}) or as a percentage of $\dot{V}O_2max$, if measured. Patients usually understand HR_{max} better than the concept of $\dot{V}O_2max$, which is why $HR_{exer\,tr}$ is the preferred value. For example, the formula for $HR_{exer\,tr}$ using a straight percentage such as 60% of the patient's HR_{max} would be as follows: $HR_{exer\,tr} = 0.6 \times HR_{max}$.

If the patient's cardiac reserve is taken into consideration when deriving $HR_{exer\,tr}$, the intensity of effort is derived by first subtracting the patient's resting (true basal) heart rate (HR_{rest}) from the HR_{max} obtained during an exercise stress test. If a patient does not undergo an exercise stress test, HR_{max} can be estimated by subtracting her or his age from the value 220. Use caution with this generalized approach to determining HR_{max} for an individual; an age-predicted HR_{max} based on healthy individuals may not be truly applicable because individuals with NIDDM may have lower HR_{max} at maximal effort (Lampman et al., 1987; Schneider, Khachadurian, Amorosa, Clemow, & Ruderman, 1992). The difference between HR_{max} and HR_{rest} is the patient's heart rate reserve ($HR_{reserve}$). $HR_{reserve}$ is then multiplied by 40% to 90%, depending subjectively on the patient's initial level of fitness as determined during screening and treadmill performance, to give a value that is added to the HR_{rest}. $HR_{reserve}$ plus HR_{rest} is the heart rate ($HR_{exer\,tr}$) that the patient should maintain during aerobic exercise training sessions. For example, to calculate a $HR_{exer\,tr}$ using a 60% intensity of effort level, the formula is as follows:

$$HR_{exer\,tr} = 60\% \ (HR_{max} - HR_{rest}) + HR_{rest}$$

Examples of both methods for a patient with a HR_{rest} of 80 beats per min and a HR_{max} of 160 beats per min are as follows:

1. Straight Percentage

$$
\begin{aligned}
HR_{exer\,tr} &= 60\% \times HR_{max} \\
&= 0.6 \times 160 \\
&= 96 \text{ beats/min}
\end{aligned}
$$

2. Heart Rate Reserve and Percentage

$$
\begin{aligned}
HR_{exer\,tr} &= 60\% \ (HR_{max} - HR_{rest}) + HR_{rest} \\
&= 0.6 \ (160 - 80) + 80 \\
&= 48 + 80 \\
&= 128 \text{ beats/min}
\end{aligned}
$$

As shown, using the $HR_{reserve}$ formula as compared with using a straight percentage results in a higher $HR_{exer\ tr}$ for the same HR_{rest} and HR_{max}. If the patient is extremely deconditioned and has significant coronary artery disease or any other major debilitating disease, adding 20 HR beats to the HR_{rest} results gives an adequate initial $HR_{exer\ tr}$ for embarking on an exercise program.

The best approach to establish training intensity during the early stages of exercise training that will allow the patient to build stamina is to use a low percentage, such as 40% to 50%, to establish a target heart rate (Lampman & Schteingart, 1991; Lampman, 1987). $HR_{exer\ tr}$ should be maintained within ± 5 beats per min through the exercise session. Intensity of effort should be strenuous enough to optimally improve the patient's cardiorespiratory function (Paffenbarger, Wing, & Hyde, 1978; Slattery, Jacobs, & Nachman, 1989), but not so vigorous as to place the individual at an increased risk for cardiovascular complications, musculoskeletal injuries, or both. As a person's fitness level improves and muscles become stronger, a higher percentage (60% to 75%) can be used to increase training effort, although patients with many advanced disease complications should stay at the low-intensity level throughout their entire exercise training programs. As a patient becomes better trained, bradycardia, a subtle mechanism by which the exercise effort is increased as a patient achieves the $HR_{exer\ tr,}$ should occur.

As the intensity of exercise increases, the potential for orthopedic and vascular complications also increases. If this is a concern, then a low intensity (e.g., 50% HR_{max} or less) can be maintained throughout the patient's entire program. This approach can still be beneficial for improving cardiorespiratory function, especially if exercise training progress is accomplished through increasing the duration of effort as discussed below.

Because the cardiorespiratory response to exercise requires approximately 2.5 to 3 min to plateau or reach a relatively steady state, the patient should measure heart rate after 3 min or longer while exercising. Exercise intensity can be monitored by measuring the heart rate (pulse) response to exercise at one of three different anatomical sites:

- Wrist on thumb side (radial pulse)
- Side of neck next to windpipe (carotid pulse)
- Left side of chest for actual heart beat

The pulse should be checked before starting the exercise session, during the warm-up period, while exercising, and following exercise during the cool-down period. Because the heart rate decelerates quickly after stopping exercise, the pulse should be counted for 10 or 15 sec immediately after cessation of exercise. The count should begin on a full beat while timing with a wristwatch, stopwatch, or wall clock. If the count does not end on an even beat, add a half beat to the count. Multiplying the 10-sec count by 6 or the 15-sec count by 4 will give the $HR_{exer\ tr}$ in beats per min. The patient should continue to slowly step in place, walk slowly, or move the legs slowly if exercising on an exercise apparatus while measuring the heart rate response. This mild muscle action (muscle pump) following vigorous exercise will help prevent pooling of blood in the legs, a situation that may cause a patient to feel lightheaded.

By periodically measuring the $HR_{exer\ tr}$, the patient can closely control exercise intensity throughout the exercise training session. Special electronic devices accurately measure heart rate response, but they are fairly expensive. Before purchasing a heart rate measuring device, the patient should make sure the instrument is accurate and can be easily read while exercising.

Some patients, especially the elderly, are unable to measure their pulse accurately. In this case, the intensity can be grossly determined by the patient's perceived feelings of exertion (rate of perceived exertion or RPE). The RPE should range between easy to mild at first and can progress to moderate to slightly hard depending on the patient's abilities and medical condition. Individuals who are checking their $HR_{exer\ tr}$ responses directly may also find it easy to maintain the exercise intensity by RPE as they become familiar with their physiological responses to exercise.

Duration of Exercise

When initially embarking on an exercise program, patients should take a low-intensity, longer-duration approach to accomplishing a total amount of energy expenditure. This approach should allow for musculoskeletal adaptations and minimize the risk for orthopedic and cardiac problems. The recommended duration of exercise effort for improving and maintaining a sufficient level of physical fitness is in the range of 30 to 60 min. Because it is initially difficult for most patients to sustain activity for this long, the recommended total workout can be accomplished through intermittent bouts of exercise (e.g., fast walking) lasting from 2 to 10 min, interspersed with periods of reduced activity (e.g., slow walking) for 1 to 2 min. Adding these intermittent bouts of peak intensity (reaching $HR_{exer\ tr}$) should equal 30 to 60 min of exercise.

Progression of Effort

Patients will notice physical and physiological changes shortly after embarking on an exercise training program, and they should be able to exercise more easily at their recommended exercise intensity for a longer exercise duration. As these adaptations to training occur, patients should concentrate on improving their endurance rather than increasing their intensity until their muscles have become well-conditioned to efficiently handle the work. It is best initially to alter the duration of exercise rather than the intensity of effort. If a patient progresses normally, he or she may alter workouts by varying the intensity or duration of effort (or both). A prudent approach, if a patient is able to reach a markedly greater effort while training, is to have the patient repeat another treadmill test. In general, a patient's total work effort should progress slowly during the first 3 to 5 weeks (i.e., 1-2 min per session), progress more rapidly after 6 to 16 weeks, and reach maintenance by 17 to 24 weeks. Highly competitive activities should not occur for the beginner until after 18 to 24 weeks of basic exercise preparation.

Frequency of Training

Exercising on a regular basis, at least three to five sessions per week, is the best approach to training. Exercise can easily be performed daily, especially if different activities are chosen each day. Alternating modes of activity will recruit different muscle groups when exercising routinely and should help prevent overuse injuries. Patients on insulin therapy should exercise daily to balance daily insulin and caloric needs. Obese patients should exercise 5 to 7 days weekly for optimizing weight loss (Lampman & Schteingart, 1991; Stern, Titchenal, & Johnson, 1987).

Injury Prevention and Safety Considerations

The potential for muscular-skeletal injuries always exists when participating in any exercise program. It is important to set realistic goals for patients because abrupt increases in the intensity or duration of exercise are major factors leading to cardiac, muscular, skeletal, and joint injuries, and possibly to metabolic problems such as proteinuria. During an exercise session, patients can help avoid injuries by warming up thoroughly and stretching, and by gradually increasing intensity to reach their assigned $HR_{exer\ tr}$. Patients should cool down slowly after completing their exercise sessions and should always take the time to stretch their muscles during the cool-down period. Orthopedic complications are usually minor, but they can result in major medical problems if ignored. If the patient develops persistent minor muscle or joint pain, he or she should rest these areas for a few days.

Metabolic Control

It is preferable to wait 1 to 2 hr after a meal before exercising. A patient on insulin therapy should never exercise when blood insulin concentrations are at their peak. Insulin should be injected subcutaneously over a nonexercising muscle. Patients should only exercise when in good metabolic control. Patients on insulin therapy should not exercise if their blood sugars are below 120 mg/dl or above 250 mg/dl. Blood glucose monitoring, if possible, should also be performed during and after exercising to prevent hypoglycemia (Ruderman & Schneider, 1986). A patient's metabolic rate may be increased up to 14 hr after strenuous exercise, making it important to monitor postexercise blood glucose levels. Hypoglycemia is usually not a problem when patients are taking sulfonylureas, but precautionary glucose monitoring should be performed (Kemmer, Tacken, & Berger, 1987). Alcoholic beverages prior to or directly after exercising should be avoided.

Environmental Considerations, Attire, and Shoes

In general, patients with diabetes should not exercise in extreme environmental conditions of heat or cold. Shopping malls are excellent places to walk because they are environmentally controlled and usually have special programs to encourage people to exercise in social settings.

Because body temperature is maintained by evaporation of sweat, patients should wear loose-fitting, lightweight clothing while exercising. Hot and humid weather limits evaporation, so it is best to have patients exercise during the coolest parts of the day or in an air-conditioned environment and consume water before, during, and following exercise to prevent dehydration. The routine use of salt tablets or supplemental drinks containing electrolytes is not necessary unless profuse sweating occurs. A patient may have to decrease the duration or intensity of the workout during periods of extreme heat.

During cold weather, a patient needs to dress warmly by wearing several layers of clothing so a jacket or sweater can be removed if he or she becomes uncomfortably warm. Cotton or polypropylene/cotton-blend materials are best as an inner layer to absorb and transfer sweat away from the body. A nylon or polyester-blend jacket is best for an outer layer to help break the wind. Because much body heat is lost from the head, a patient should wear a ski hat that covers the ears as well as the head. Patients should wear mittens because they keep hands warmer than gloves. A patient may wear a face mask to prevent breathing cold air and the resulting vasoconstriction. If it is extremely cold, patients should exercise in indoor facilities, such as a shopping center, a school gymnasium, a YMCA, or a commercial facility.

Patients should select any major brand of running shoe or walking shoe with a built-up heel to absorb the impact of the heel striking the ground. The shoe should have a firm, but not rigid, arch support in the insole to prevent excessive pronation. Shoes with midsoles containing air or silica gel are more absorbent in reducing shearing forces at impact with the ground and should help reduce problems for individuals with peripheral neuropathy or microvascular disease. Patients should avoid tube socks because they often fold in the shoe, causing blisters. A cotton/polyester-blend stocking with a constructed toe and heel design is best to prevent these problems. Patients should inspect their feet before and after they exercise.

Exercise Equipment

Emphasize good exercise attire and shoes prior to considering the purchase of special exercise equipment such as weights, step climbers, rowing machines, treadmills, stationary, road, or trail bicycles, and so on. Certain equipment is very useful and can have a major impact on a patient's adherence to a training program if it is used routinely and properly. As a general guideline for purchasing equipment, the patient should remember the following:

- Never buy on impulse.
- Thoroughly study the purpose of the machine and what muscle groups it conditions.
- Consult with people who have similar equipment.
- Review consumer and trade reports.
- Compare prices at different stores.
- Consider equipment that accommodates various body statures so friends and family members can also use the device.

Clinical Applications

The American Diabetes Association (1990) recommends that exercise training play an integral role in therapy of patients with diabetes. In studies of people with Type II diabetes mellitus physical training posed no major complications in subjects (Krotkiewski et al., 1985; Schneider et al., 1992), yet its use has been limited and concerns about exercise persist (National Institutes of Health, 1987). Patients with poor circulatory responses due to ischemia, diabetic retinopathy, and the tendency to be hypoglycemic may still exercise safely if its intensity results in a moderate blood pressure response (Bernbaum, Albert, Cohen, & Drimmer, 1989). The best approach is to have patients participate in exercise programs involving longer duration of moderate effort. Individuals with special needs can usually engage in exercise training programs successfully with this approach (Lampman et al., 1987).

Model Treatment Programs

Schneider, Khachadurian, Amorosa, Clemow, & Ruderman (1992) recently reported their 10-year experience with 255 diabetic patients (200 were NIDDM) in a clinical treatment program that emphasized outpatient aerobic exercise. They found advanced ischemic heart disease at baseline for 11% of the patients with Type II diabetes, and these patients were excluded from participating in the program. Patients with Type II diabetes had higher body weights, body mass index, and plasma triglycerides and lower HDL cholesterol levels than people with Type I diabetes and controls. Plasma glucose and HbA$_{1c}$ concentrations were similar in all groups. As Lampman et al. (1987) reported earlier, patients with Type II diabetes showed lower than normal $\dot{V}O_2$max at baseline. Other reports have also noted lower than normal $\dot{V}O_2$max values in patients with NIDDM and that these lower maximum aerobic levels were independent of autonomic dysfunction (Bogardus, Ravussin, Robbins, Wolfe, Horton, & Sims, 1984; National Institutes of Health, 1987; Rubler, 1981; Ruderman, Ganda, & Johansen, 1979; Saltin, Lindgarde, Lithell, Eriksso, & Gad, 1980; Schneider, Amorosa, Khachadurian, & Ruderman, 1984). Schneider et al. (1992) reported that patients participating in their model exercise program showed a marked improvement in $\dot{V}O_2$max but that the $\dot{V}O_2$max achieved was still less than what untrained sedentary controls reached. Lampman et al. (1987) reported previously that patients with NIDDM showed improvement in $\dot{V}O_2$max following 9 weeks of exercise training but not to the extent that patients without diabetes achieved. Schneider et al. (1992) further reported that a slight drop in body weight and body mass index occurred in patients with Type II diabetes. Significant reductions in fasting plasma glucose, HbA$_{1c}$, and triglyceride levels occurred in patients with Type II diabetes, but HDL cholesterol concentrations remained unchanged. Because insulin levels were unchanged, but glycemic control was improved following exercise training, the investigators suggested enhanced sensitivity to insulin. Resting blood pressure following the 3-month training program decreased slightly, as did blood pressure responses to submaximal exercise.

An important aspect of this lifestyle modification program was the compliance of the patients. Most complied with this formal exercise program well over the initial 6 weeks, but drop-outs reached 50% by 3 months, and by 1 year only 10% of the patients remained in the formal exercise program. However, most of the drop-outs continued to exercise on their own at least twice a week. Self-referred rather than physician-referred patients were more likely to comply long term. As previously reported (Haynes, 1976), long-term compliance was improved if a patient's spouse strongly supported the program.

Heath, Leonard, Wlson, Kendrick, and Powell (1987) studied the benefits of exercise training in the Zuni Indians of New Mexico (a population with a high incidence of Type II diabetes). Fifty-six nonparticipants with NIDDM were matched by age, sex, health care provider, and duration of NIDDM to individuals participating in a formal community exercise program. Those undergoing exercise training had a mean weight loss of 4 kg, whereas those not exercising had a mean loss of 0.9 kg. Exercise training resulted in a mean drop of 43 mg/dl in fasting blood glucose levels, compared to only a mean drop of 2 mg/dl in the nonparticipating controls. Most subjects undergoing exercise training were able to stop their hypoglycemic medication. A follow-up report further substantiated that diabetes risk reduction and glycemic control in Zuni Indians can be obtained through a community-based exercise and weight control program (Heath, Wilson, Smith & Leonard, 1991).

Managing Patients With Special Needs

Bernbaum, Albert, & Cohen (1989) studied 29 individuals with diabetes-related retinopathy and blindness. Each subject was evaluated for cardio-vascular autonomic function and exercise tolerance before entering an exercise rehabilitation program. Inadequate chronotropic responses were observed in 28 patients, abnormal heart rate responses to postural maneuvers were observed in 23 patients, and postural hypertension was observed in 9 patients. Following exercise training, blood glucose decreased by a mean of 76 ± 9 mg/dl after each exercise session even though mild-intensity exercise was performed.

Changes in lipids, body weight, and blood pressure during pregnancy were examined in 312 diabetic women and 356 control women starting within 21 days after conception (Peterson et al., 1992). Cholesterol levels increased, although not to abnormal levels, in all subjects, but they remained significantly lower in the diabetic women at 12 weeks. Triglyceride levels remained normal in both groups until 10 weeks, when they became lower in the diabetic women. No body weight differences were noted between groups at baseline, but the diabetic group gained a significantly greater body weight between 6 and 8 weeks. The nondiabetic women maintained their systolic blood pressures, whereas systolic blood pressures increased in the diabetic patients. These results suggest the importance of maintaining good diet and exercise programs during gestation to reduce the risk for long-term cardiovascular disease.

Jovanovic-Peterson, Durak, and Peterson (1989) studied the impact of physical training on glucose tolerance in 19 women with gestational diabetes mellitus. Patients were randomly assigned to receive either a 6-week diet program alone or diet plus exercise. Exercise involved arm ergometry training six times a week for 6 weeks. After the study, glycosylated hemoglobin values were lower for the group that exercised as compared to the group that used diet alone. Final fasting glucoses were 87.6 $\pm$ 6.2 mg/dl for the diet group as compared with the results for the exercise plus diet group, 70.1 $\pm$ 6.6 mg/dl. Furthermore, the exercise group showed lower 1-hour plasma glucose levels—187.5 $\pm$ 12.9 mg/dl for the diet alone group and 105.9 $\pm$ 18.9 mg/dl for the exercise plus diet group.

Case Studies

The following are typical case studies of patients receiving exercise therapy.

▬▬▬ CASE STUDY 1

A 42-year-old obese female presented to the clinic with known Type II diabetes for 10 years. Her initial body weight was 310 lb. She had gained this weight since delivering her second child at age 20. She underwent an exercise stress test with the speed set at 3 mi per hr with increments in grade of 3% every 3 min. Her resting heart rate was 82 beats per min. She reached a heart rate response of 168 beats per min at peak exercise. The test was stopped due to leg fatigue. Her EKG tracing was normal at rest and showed no ST-T segment changes or arrhythmias with exercise. The patient denied angina pectoris during exercise. She had no orthopedic problems that would prevent her from engaging in a mild exercise program or history of osteoarthritis, rheumatoid arthritis, neuropathy, or retinopathy.

The patient was given an intermittent exercise program of walking and stationary cycling. She was to exercise on a daily basis. Her $HR_{exer\ tr}$ was established at 125 beats per min with a range of 120 to 130 beats per min. Intermittent exercise consisting of 3- to 5-min bouts followed by a 1- to 2-min recovery period (with reduced intensity of effort) was established. The exercise/recovery bouts were to be repeated at least 6 to 15 times to ensure 30 min of exercise per exercise session. Prior to and following exercise the patient was instructed to perform low-intensity exercise as warm-up and cool-down, respectively. Progression was to be achieved by increasing her exercise bouts by 1 min per week. A 1,500 calorie diabetic diet was prescribed.

The patient did well with her program and markedly improved her functional capacity from 18 ml/kg/min to 35 ml/kg/min. She improved her physical fitness level to the point that she was performing mild jogging for most of her exercise session. She lost 170 lb in approximately 50 weeks. She eventually added a variety of other activities such as aerobic dance, stair climbing, using a cross country ski machine, resistance training, and the like to supplement her initial program. She acknowledged feeling much better, having more energy, sleeping more soundly for fewer hours, and having more stamina for activities of daily living.

Her blood chemistry changes during her exercise program were as follows:

Measure	Changes
• Glucose (mg/dl)	210 to 104
• Insulin (μu/ml)	18 to 6
• Total Cholesterol (mg/dl)	263 to 202
• HDL cholesterol (mg/dl)	28 to 41
• LDL cholesterol (mg/dl)	148 to 128
• Triglycerides (mg/dl)	435 to 166

■■■■■■   **CASE STUDY 2**

A 68-year-old male with Type II diabetes and peripheral vascular occlusive arterial disease resulting in significant intermittent claudication was placed on a mild-intensity exercise program. His baseline weight was 215 pounds. His major risk factors for atherosclerotic vascular disease included a history of heavy cigarette smoking, 25 years of known diabetes treated currently with insulin (50 μu/ml/day), mild hypertension (148/85 mmHg), hypertriglyceridemia (235 mg/dl), and hypercholesterolemia (252 mg/dl). He had known coronary artery disease and mild diabetic neuropathy.

The patient underwent an exercise tolerance stress test, which was stopped due to severe intermittent claudication of the left leg greater than in the right leg. A peak pressure rate product of 265 (peak: HR = 134 b/min and BP = 198 mmHg) was reached. No myocardial ischemia as detected by ST-T changes was noted on the ECG during exercise.

Intermittent exercise of walking and stationary cycling was prescribed. The patient was encouraged, however, to choose walking as often as possible to improve metabolism in the gastrocemius and soleus muscles. The patient was told to use short strides so as not to restrict forward motion. Exercise bouts were initially set for 2 to 3 min followed by a 1- to 2-min recovery period. The patient was instructed to extend himself beyond the point of fairly severe intermittent claudication pain but to immediately stop exercising if he experienced angina pectoris. The exercise-recovery cycle was to be repeated 10 to 20 times to ensure at least 30 min of exercise per training session. If performed by cycling, the recovery period was to be walking slowly around the room. Progression was to be accomplished by increasing the bouts by 1 min per week. Because intermittent claudication due to his advanced peripheral vascular disease (PVD), rather than cardiac dysfunction, limited his exercise performance, the patient was not instructed to monitor closely his exercise heart rate response.

The patient was advised to exercise in a pair of walking or jogging shoes with an absorbing midsole composition of air or silica gel to reduce shearing forces at heel strike. Moreover, he was advised to replace his shoe insoles with special arch-supporting insoles to prevent excessive pronation. He was instructed to check his blood glucose levels before, during, and after exercise and to check his feet before and after exercise for abrasions or blisters.

The patient markedly increased his ability to ambulate, walking only one block initially to later walking continuously for 30 min. At a fast pace, he still developed calf pain, but his routine speed of ambulation drastically improved. The patient's insulin needs were reduced by 34%. He felt better, had more stamina, and had fewer symptoms related to PVD. He denied experiencing any cardiac problems throughout his exercise training program.

The patient's blood chemistry changes during exercise therapy were as follows:

Measure	Changes
• Fasting Glucose (mg/dl)	250 to 128
• Fasting Insulin (μu/ml)	24 to 15
• Total Cholesterol (mg/dl)	252 to 220
• HDL cholesterol (mg/dl)	32 to 38
• LDL cholesterol (mg/dl)	162 to 135
• Triglycerides (mg/dl)	235 to 170

References

American College of Sports Medicine. (1991). *Guidelines for exercise testing and prescription.* Philadelphia: Lea & Febiger.

American Diabetes Association. (1990). Position statement: Diabetes mellitus and exercise. *Diabetes Care,* **13,** 805.

Bergstrom, R.W., Newell-Morris, L.L., Leonetti, D.L., Shuman, W.P., Wahl, P.W., & Fujimoto, W.Y. (1990). Association of elevated fasting C-peptide level and increased intra-abdominal fat distribution with development of NIDDM in Japanese-American men. *Diabetes,* **39,** 104-111.

Bernbaum, M., Albert, S.G., & Cohen, J.D. (1989). Exercise training in individuals with diabetes retinopathy and blindness. *Archives of Physical Medicine and Rehabilitation,* **70**(8), 605-611.

Bernbaum, M., Albert, S.G., Cohen, J.D., & Drimmer, A. (1989). Cardiovascular conditioning in individuals with diabetic retinopathy. *Diabetes Care,* **12,** 740-741.

Bogardus, C., Ravussin, E., Robbins, D.C., Wolfe, R.R., Horton, E.S., & Sims, E.A.H. (1984). Effects of physical training and diet therapy on carbohydrate metabolism in patients with glucose intolerance and noninsulin dependent diabetes mellitus. *Diabetes,* **33,** 311-318.

Durak, E.P., Jovanovic-Peterson, L., & Peterson, C.M. (1990). Randomized crossover study of effect of resistance training on glycemic control, muscular strength, and cholesterol in Type I diabetic men. *Diabetes Care,* **13,** 1039-1043.

Goldberg, A.P. (1989). Aerobic and resistive exercise modify risk factors for coronary heart disease. *Medicine and Science in Sports and Exercise,* **21,** 669-674.

Haynes, R.B. (1976). A critical review of "determinant" of patient compliance with therapeutic regimen. In D.L. Sackett & R.B. Haynes (Eds.), *Compliance with therapeutic regimens* (p. 40). Baltimore: Johns Hopkins University.

Heath, G.W., Leonard, B.E., Wilson, R.H., Kendrick, J.S., & Powell, K.E. (1987). Community-based exercise intervention: Zuni Diabetes Project. *Diabetes Care, 10*(4), 579-583.

Heath, G.W., Wilson, R.H., Smith, J., & Leonard, B.E. (1991). Community-based exercise and weight control: Diabetes risk reduction and glycemic control in Zuni Indians. *American Journal of Clinical Nutrition, 53*(Suppl. 6), 1642S-1646S.

Jovanovic-Peterson, L., Durak, E.P., & Peterson, C.M. (1989). Randomized trial of diet versus diet plus cardiovascular conditioning on glucose levels in gestational diabetes. *American Journal of Obstetrics and Gynecology, 161*(2), 415-419.

Jovanovic-Peterson, L., & Peterson, C.M. (1991). Is exercise safe or useful for gestational diabetic women? *Diabetes, 40*(Suppl. 2), 179-181.

Kemmer, F.W., Tacken, M., & Berger, M. (1987). Mechanism of exercise-induced hypoglycemia during sulfonylurea treatment. *Diabetes, 36,* 1178-1182.

King, H., & Kriska, A.M. (1992). Prevention of Type II diabetes by physical training: Epidemiological considerations and study methods. *Diabetes Care, 15*(Suppl. 11), 1794-1799.

Krotkiewski, M., Loaroth, P., Manrwoukas, K., Wroblewski, Z., Rebuffe-Serive, M., Holme, G., Smith, N., & Bjorntorp, P. (1985). Effects of physical training on insulin secretion and effectiveness and glucose metabolism in obesity and Type II diabetes (noninsulin dependent) in diabetes mellitus. *Diabetologia, 28,* 881-890.

Lampman, R.M. (1987). Evaluating and prescribing exercise for elderly patients. *Geriatrics, 42,* 63-76.

Lampman, R.M., & Schteingart, D.E. (1991). Effects of exercise on glucose control, lipid metabolism, and insulin sensitivity in hypertriglyceridemia and non-insulin dependent diabetes mellitus. *Medicine and Science in Sports and Exercise, 23*(6), 703-712.

Lampman, R.M., Schteingart, D.E., Santinga, J.T., Savage, P.J., Hydrick, C.R., Bassett, D.R., & Block, W.D. (1987). The influence of physical training on glucose tolerance, insulin sensitivity, and lipid and lipoprotein concentrations in middle-aged hypertriglyceridemia, carbohydrate intolerant men. *Diabetologia, 30,* 380-385.

Lillioja, S., & Bogardus, C. (1988). Obesity and insulin resistance: Lessons learned from the Pima Indians. *Diabetes and Metabolism Review, 4,* 517-540.

Miller, W.J., Sherman, W.M., & Ivy, J.L. (1984). Effect of strength training on glucose tolerance and post-glucose insulin response. *Medicine and Science in Sports and Exercise, 16,* 539-543.

National Institutes of Health. (1987). Consensus development conference on diet and exercise in non-insulin dependent diabetes mellitus. *Diabetes Care, 10,* 639-644.

Ohlson, L.O., Larsson, B., Suardsud, K., Welin, L., Eriksson, H., Wilhelmsen, R., Bjorntorp, P., & Tibblin, G. (1985). The influence of body fat distribution on the incidence of diabetes mellitus 13.5 years of follow-up of the participants in the study of men born in 1913. *Diabetes,* **34,** 1055-1058.

Paffenbarger, R.S., Wing, A.L., & Hyde, R.T. (1978). Physical activity as an index of heart attack risk in college alumni. *American Journal of Epidemiology,* **108,** 161-175.

Peterson, C.M., Jovanovic-Peterson, L., Mills, J.L., Conley, M.R., Knopp, R.H., Reed, G.F., Aarons, J.H., Holmes, L.B., Brown, Z., Van Allen, M., et al. (1992). The diabetes in early pregnancy study: Changes in cholesterol, triglycerides, body weight, and blood pressure. The National Institute of Child Health and Human Development—the diabetes in early pregnancy study. *American Journal of Obstetrics and Gynecology,* **166**(2), 513-518.

Reaven, G.M. (1988). Banting lecture: Role of insulin resistance in human diabetes. *Diabetes,* **37,** 1595-1607.

Rubler, S. (1981). Asymptomatic diabetic females: Exercise testing. *NY State Journal of Medicine,* **81,** 1185-1191.

Ruderman, N.B., Ganda, O.P., & Johansen, K. (1979). The effect of physical training on glucose tolerance and plasma lipids in maturity onset diabetes. *Diabetes,* **28**(Suppl. 1), 89-91.

Ruderman, N.B., & Haudenschild, C. (1984). Diabetes as an atherogenic factor. *Progress in Cardiovascular Disease,* **26,** 373-412.

Ruderman, N.B., & Schneider, S. (1986). Exercise and the insulin-dependent diabetic. *Hospital Practice,* **21,** 41-51.

Saltin, B., Lindgarde, F., Lithell, H., Eriksson, K.F., & Gad, P. (1980). Metabolic effects of long-term physical training in maturity onset diabetes. *Excerpta Medica Amsterdam,* **9,** 345-350.

Schneider, S.H., Amorosa, L.F., Khachadurian, A.K., & Ruderman, N.D. (1984). Studies on the mechanism of improved glucose control during regular exercise in Type 2 (noninsulin dependent) diabetes. *Diabetologia,* **26,** 355-360.

Schneider, S.H., Khachadurian, A.K., Amorosa, L.F., Clemow, L., & Ruderman, N.B. (1992). Ten-year experience with an exercise-based outpatient life-style modification program in the treatment of diabetes mellitus. *Diabetes Care,* **15**(Suppl. 4), 1800-1810.

Slattery, M.L., Jacobs, D.R., & Nachman, M.Z. (1989). Leisure time, physical activity and coronary heart disease death. *Circulation,* **79,** 304-311.

Stern, J.S., Titchenal, C.A., & Johnson, P.R. (1987). Obesity: Does exercise make a difference? In A. Howard (Ed.), *Recent Advances in Obesity Research* (pp. 337-349). London: Newman.

Warram, J.H., Martin, B.C., Krolewski, A.S., Soeldner, J.S., & Kahn, C.R. (1990). Slow glucose removal rate and hyperinsulinemia precede the development of Type II diabetes in offspring with diabetic parents. *Annuals of Internal Medicine,* **190,** 909-915.

Yki-Järvinen, H., & Koivisto, V.A. (1983). Effects of body composition on insulin sensitivity. *Diabetes,* **32,** 965-969.

Glossary

acidosis—Abnormal state of increased acidity in the body due to rapid and incomplete breakdown of fat.

autoimmune—A condition in which antibodies are produced against the body's own tissues that may result in autoimmune diseases.

autoimmunity—A condition in which specific humoral or cell-mediated immune responses occur against constituents of the body's own tissues.

background retinopathy—Early stages of retinopathy associated with diabetes mellitus; it is progressively characterized by microaneurysms, intraretinal punctate hemorrhages, yellow, waxy exudates, cotton-wool patches, and neovascularization of the retinal and optic disk, which may project into the vitreous proliferation of fibrous tissue, vitreous hemorrhage, and retinal detachment.

basal—Baseline or resting, pertaining here to levels before exercise.

basement membrane—Basal lamina or basement lamina, a membranous structure characterized by its ultrastructure and localization and topographically characterized as extracellular and always located in close opposition to a cell surface. In most cases it forms a sheath between the cell and the interstitial space, except in the glomerular capillaries and the central nervous system, where the membrane is delineated by cells on both sides. Vascular system basement membranes are prominent.

beta cell—Cells of the Islets of Langerhans of the pancreas that secrete insulin.

C-peptide—The connecting peptide chain that is removed during the cleavage of proinsulin to insulin. When secreted in association with insulin, indicates some residual beta cell function in diabetes.

catecholamines (epinephrine and norepinephrine)—Biologically active amines that produce marked effects on the nervous system and cardiovascular system, metabolic rate, temperature, and smooth muscle.

cortisol—A glucocorticoid secreted by the adrenal medulla. Cortisol plays an important role in the utilization of carbohydrate, protein, and fat. About 95% of all glucocorticoid activity results from cortisol secretion.

counterregulation—The production of glucose by the liver, stimulated by the counterregulatory hormones (e.g., epinephrine, cortisol, glucagon, growth hormone).

depancreatized—To deprive of the pancreas, as with surgical removal.

diabetes mellitus—The full name of the disease commonly known as diabetes. In Greek, the word *diabetes* means "passing through," and in Latin *mellitus* means "honey," describing the presence of sugar in the urine.

downregulation—A decrease in the number of insulin receptors at the surface of the cell membrane in response to high circulating levels of insulin.

erythrocyte—A mature red blood cell.

euglycemic—Near normal blood glucose level.

free fatty acid—The basic lipid component of both triglycerides and phospholipids. These long-chain hydrocarbon organic acids are used to provide energy for metabolic processes and other intracellular functions.

free insulin—Insulin that is not antibody bound. When insulin is given exogenously in diabetes, the body produces antibodies that may attach to it. The insulin that is not bound by antibodies is called free insulin.

glucagon—A hormone produced and secreted by the alpha cells of the pancreas with the capability of influencing liver production of glucose.

gluconeogenesis—see glyconeogenesis.

glucose clamp—A technique in which glucose and insulin are given simultaneously to achieve a desired blood glucose level (e.g., 90 ± 10 mg/dl) for a specific period of time. The glucose clamp is used to determine total body insulin sensitivity.

glucosuria—Abnormal amount of glucose in the urine.

glycemic excursions—Large variations in blood glucose.

glycemic response—The rise or fall in blood glucose that is caused by something, for example, exercise, a meal, or stress.

glycemic state—Referring to blood glucose level.

glycogen—The form of stored carbohydrate in the body tissues (e.g., liver, muscle) for future conversion to glucose for performing work or releasing heat.

glycogenesis—The formation or synthesis of glycogen.

glycolysis—Conversion of glycogen to glucose.

glycolytic—Pertaining to hydrolyzing glucose.

glyconeogenesis—The formation of carbohydrate from noncarbohydrate sources (e.g., fatty acids, amino acids).

glycosylation—Formation of linkages between various tissues or proteins and glycosyl groups in diabetes.

growth hormone—Any substance that stimulates growth, especially one secreted by the anterior pituitary gland, which controls the rate of skeletal and visceral growth and directly affects protein, carbohydrate, and lipid metabolism.

hemoglobin A$_{1c}$—Portion of the hemoglobin molecule bound with glucose. In general, normal levels may range from 4% to 6%, depending on the laboratory. Hemoglobin A$_{1c}$ is a more specific form of hemoglobin A$_1$. The levels of HbA$_{1c}$ are usually 2% to 3% lower than HbA$_1$.

histocompatibility antigen—A system of antigens that can stimulate an immune response leading to rejection of a specific tissue.

"honeymoon" phase—A period of time occurring shortly after diagnosis of Type I diabetes during which the disease appears to be in remission. During this time, some residual beta cell function occurs and low levels of insulin are produced.

hyperglycemia—A blood glucose level above normal (i.e., greater than 90 ± 10 mg/dl). In the presence of diabetes hyperglycemia may be defined as a fasting blood glucose greater than 140 mg/dl.

hypoglycemia—A blood glucose level below normal (i.e., less than 90 mg/dl ± 10 mg/dl). In diabetes the symptoms of hypoglycemia may be related to the absolute level of blood glucose or the rate of decrease in blood glucose. Symptoms of hypoglycemia include cold sweats, pallor, trembling, confusion, irritability, headache, drowsiness, dizziness, heart palpitations, weakness, nausea, and blurred vision.

insulin—A hormone produced by the beta cells of the pancreas. Insulin is essential for the proper maintenance of food utilization and blood glucose levels.

insulin "pump"—A means of administering subcutaneous insulin on a continuous basis that is usually worn at the waist to deliver insulin abdominally.

intracellular membrane—A membrane occurring or situated within a cell; the inner membrane of the cell.

intramuscular—taking place within the muscle.

intrinsic—Situated or occurring within.

isoform—Multiple forms of a given biological substance within a single species of organism. Glucose transporters are present in several isoforms within mammalian muscle and adipocytes (e.g., Glut 1, Glut 4).

ketoacidosis—Acidosis accompanied by ketosis (see ketosis).

ketones—Substances formed in the breakdown of fat. The presence of ketones is evidence of incomplete utilization of large amounts of fat.

ketosis—The accumulation in the body of ketones, resulting from the incomplete metabolism of fatty acids, that is generally caused by carbohydrate deficiency or inadequate utilization. See acidosis.

lactate—A salt of lactic acid that is the metabolic end product of glycolysis, can provide energy anaerobically in skeletal muscle during heavy exercise, and can be oxidized in the heart aerobically for energy or converted back to glucose in the liver.

macrovascular—Pertaining to the large vessels, for example, macrovascular complications.

microangiopathy—A diabetic vascular disease of the small vessels that leads to diabetic retinopathy and nephropathy.

microvascular—Pertaining to the small vessels (less than 100 microns), for example, microvascular complications.

monocyte—A blood cell, the largest of the cells in the normal blood, with a round, oval, or indented nucleus.

nephropathy—Disease of the kidneys that may involve the glomeruli or tubules of the nephrons in diabetes.

neuroarthropathy—A joint disease (as Charcot's joint) that is associated with a disorder of the nervous system.

neuropathy—In general, functional disturbances, pathological changes, or both in the peripheral nervous system. Particularly in diabetes, neuropathy involves a segmental demyelination of the peripheral nerves. It also involves a chronic symmetrical sensory polyneuropathy affecting first the nerves of the lower limbs and often the autonomic nerves.

pancreas—An endocrine gland located behind the stomach that produces insulin, glucagon, and other substances important in digestion.

pharmacokinetics—The action of drugs or pharmacologic agents in the body, including absorption, distribution, localization in tissues, biotransformation, and excretion.

portal—The entrance for blood entering the liver.

postabsorptive—Following digestion of a meal.

postprandial—Following the eating of a meal.

precursor—A forerunner of something else; a substance from which another substance, usually a more biologically mature one, is formed.

preproliferative retinopathy—The second stage of retinopathy preceding proliferative retinopathy

proliferative retinopathy—Retinopathy that is fully developed and progressive.

proteinuria—Protein (usually in the form of albumin) in the urine, usually indicative of kidney damage.

pyruvate dehydrogenase—The first enzyme involved in pyruvate utilization. The pyruvate dehydrogenase complex converts pyruvate to acetyl-Co-A.

retinopathy—Changes in the retina that occur commonly with diabetes in three stages. In the early stage, background retinopathy, microaneurysms are present; in preproliferative retinopathy hemorrhaging occurs;

and in proliferative retinopathy, the final stage, fibrosis occurs, which can result in retinal detachment.

sarcolemma—The delicate elastic sheath that surrounds every striated muscle fiber.

somatostatin—A hormone that inhibits the release of somatotropin; also, a peptide released from the hypothalamus that inhibits insulin and gastrin secretion.

splanchnic—Pertaining to supplying the viscera (e.g., splanchnic vessels).

submaximal exercise—A percentage less than the maximum exercise effort an individual can perform.

unit—A standard of measurement. Insulin dosage is prescribed in units—U-100 insulin has 100 units in a cc (cubic centimeter); 1,000 units are in a 10 cc bottle.

Valsalva maneuver—A forcible exhalation against a closed glottis.

Index

A

Abelman, W.H., 38

Acute exercise, response to. *See* Response to acute exercise

Adaptation to training
  normal (without diabetes), 17-18, 115-117
  with Type I diabetes
    in blood glucose control, 61-66
    complications of diabetes and, 77-78
    in insulin sensitivity, 66-71, 72
    in lipids/lipoprotein levels, 72, 75-77
    in skeletal muscle metabolism, 72-75
  with Type II diabetes
    in adipose tissue metabolism, 123
    in blood glucose control, 118-120, 121, 129, 130
    cardiovascular disease risk and, 128-129
    diet and, 119, 121, 128-130
    in insulin secretion, 119, 120-121, 122-123
    insulin sensitivity and, 117, 121-123, 124-125, 126
    in maximal oxygen consumption, 127-128
    obesity and, 119, 126-127, 129-130
    overview of, 117-118
    in skeletal muscle metabolism, 118, 123, 126-127
    weight loss, 129-130

Adipose tissue, metabolism in, 123. *See also* Fat metabolism

Adolescents, training adaptations in, 62

Adult-onset diabetes. *See* Type II diabetes (non-insulin dependent diabetes mellitus, NIDDM)

Aerobic exercise, with Type II diabetes, 174, 180-181

Ahlborg, 43

Ala-Houhala, I., 159-160

Albert, S.G., 182

Allenberg, K., 128

Almar, A.O., 157

American Diabetes Association, 180

Amorosa, L.F., 180-181

Ananthakrishnan, P., 53

Angina, 102

Arteriosclerosis, 16, 19

Atherosclerosis
    level of risk of, 15
    lipid abnormalities and, 12
    in mortality with Type II diabetes, 5
    risk factors, and exercise with Type II diabetes, 97, 103, 128

Attire for exercise, 179-180

Autoimmune aspects of Type I diabetes, 1, 2-3

Autonomic neuropathy, 146, 154-155

B

Bak, J.F., 65, 71, 73-74

Barlow, J., 43

Barnard, R.J., 128-129
Beck-Nielsen, H., 43
Benefits of exercise
 with complications of diabetes, 152, 160
 in general, 20
 with Type I diabetes, 144-147, 152, 160
 with Type II diabetes, 169-170, 171
Berger, M., 38, 45
Bergstrom, B., 154
Bernbaum, M., 153, 182
Bjorntorp, P., 122
Blando, L., 130
Blindness, level of risk of, 15. *See also* Retinopathy
Blood glucose levels. *See* Glucose levels; Glycemic control
Blood pressure. *See also* Hypertension
 exercise response with Type II diabetes, 103-104
 exercise therapy with complications and, 158-159, 160, 161
 hypotension, 154
 training adaptations with Type II diabetes, 130, 181
Bonen, A., 43, 69, 71
Bonen, A.B., 116
Bramnert, M., 154
Brodsky, I., 41-42
Brozinick, J.T., 126
Bruce, D.G., 94
Burstein, R., 100

C

Callaham, P.R., 103
Campaigne, Barbara N., 46-48, 62
Cancer risk, 20
Capillarization. *See* Muscle capillarization in training adaptations
Cardiac metabolism, in exercise response, 103
Cardiorespiratory exercise response with Type II diabetes, 97
Cardiovascular disease risk. *See also* Atherosclerosis; Coronary artery disease
 (CAD) risk; Coronary heart disease with Type II diabetes
 exercise in general and, 19-20
 level of, with diabetes, 15
 lipid/lipoprotein abnormalities and, 13
 screening for, 140-141, 171
 training adaptation with Type II diabetes and, 128-129
Cardiovascular response to exercise
 normal (without diabetes), 18, 91
 with Type II diabetes, 101-104
Caron, D., 46
Catecholamines in exercise response
 with Type I diabetes, 35, 37, 48, 49
 with Type II diabetes, 94
 without diabetes and, 87
Cerebral stroke, 15
Charuzi, I., 100
Cherny, S., 128-129
Children, training adaptations in, 62
Chisholm, D.J., 94

Cholesterol levels. *See also* High-density lipoprotein (HDL) levels
  low-density lipoprotein (LDL) levels, 20, 75, 77, 129
  in training adaptations
    with Type I diabetes, 75, 77
    with Type II diabetes, 129
  with Type I diabetes in general, 14
  with Type II diabetes in general, 13
  very-low-density lipoprotein (VLDL), 13, 14
Chronic exercise. *See* Adaptation to training
Chronic obstructive pulmonary disease (COPD), 20
Cilmi, K.M., 154
Clinical application of exercise
  management team for, 139-140, 144, 172
  overview of, 16, 17, 20-21
  with Type I diabetes
    case studies, 162-165
    complications of diabetes and, 146, 152-162
    diet and, 147-148, 152
    follow up for, 161-162
    insulin treatment and, 148-152
    overview of, 139-140
    program design and implementation, 141-152
    risks/benefits of, 144-147, 152, 154-155, 156, 158, 160
    sample programs for, 162-165
    screening/evaluation for, 140-141, 155
    shoes for, 156, 160-161
  with Type II diabetes
    case studies, 182-185
    complications of diabetes and, 169-170, 180
    diet and, 170
    environment, attire, and shoes for, 179-180
    equipment for, 180
    insulin treatment and, 178-179
    metabolic control for, 178-179
    model programs for, 180-181
    overview of, 169-171
    prescription of exercise for, 173-178
    risks of, 172, 180
    safety considerations, 178
    screening/evaluation for, 169-170, 171-172, 173
    for special needs patients, 182
Clinical management team, 139-140, 144, 172
Clothing for exercise, 179-180
  footwear, 156, 160-161, 179-180
Cohen, J.D., 182
Colon cancer risk, 20
Compliance with exercise therapy, 181
Complications of diabetes
  exercise therapy with, 146, 152-162, 169-170, 180
  overview of, 3, 5, 14-16
  screening for, 140-141
  training adaptations with Type I diabetes and, 77-78
Continuous subcutaneous insulin infusion (CSII), 46, 48
Cool-down and warm-up, 174-175, 178

Coronary artery disease (CAD) risk
  exercise for reducing, 19
  insulin resistance and, 13
  level of, 16
  screening for, 140, 171
Coronary heart disease with Type II diabetes. *See also* Cardiovascular disease risk
  exercise response with, 102-103
  training adaptations and, 128
Cortez, M.Y., 126
Cortisol in exercise response, 87, 97
Costill, D.L., 62, 66, 72
Counterregulatory hormone response, 48, 87, 97
Cystic fibrosis, exercise benefits for, 20

D
Dahl-Jorgensen, K., 62
DeFronzo, R., 10, 98
DeFronzo, R.A., 93-94
Dehydration, 155
Devlin, J.T., 41-42, 43, 97-98, 100, 101
Diabetes. *See also* Complications of diabetes; Type I diabetes (insulin-dependent
      diabetes mellitus, IDDM); Type II diabetes (non-insulin dependent diabetes
      mellitus, NIDDM)
  gestational, 182
  medical treatment for, overview, 16-17
  physiology of, overview, 7-14
Dietary intake
  clinical applications
    in general, 16
    with Type I diabetes, 147-148, 152
    with Type II diabetes, 170
  exercise response and
    with Type I diabetes, 44, 46, 48
    with Type II diabetes, 95
  training adaptations and, with Type II diabetes, 119, 121, 128-130
Donckier, J.E., 103
Dorman, J.S., 77
Downregulation, 10
Durak, E.P., 182
Duration of exercise
  clinical applications with Type II diabetes, 173-174, 177
  exercise response and
    with Type I diabetes, 48-53
    with Type II diabetes, 94
    without diabetes, 88, 89

E
Edano, A., 130
End-stage renal disease (ESRD), 160
Endurance training, adaptations to, 18. *See also* Aerobic exercise, with Type II
      diabetes
Environment for exercise, 179
Enzymes, muscle. *See* Muscle enzymes
Epinephrine in exercise response
  with Type I diabetes, 35, 36, 37, 49, 53

with Type II diabetes, 95, 96, 97
without diabetes, 87, 89, 91
Epstein, Y., 100
Equipment for exercise, 180
Erythrocytes, insulin binding to, 71
Euglycemic clamp technique, 10, 12, 121, 122, 129, 171
Evaluation of patients. *See* Screening for exercise therapy
Exercise. *See also* Adaptation to training; Benefits of exercise; Clinical application of
    exercise; Precautions for exercise; Response to acute exercise; Risks of exercise
  with chronic disease in general, 19-20
  lack of, in risks for disease, 16
Exercise equipment, 180
Exercise prescription with Type II diabetes, 173-178. *See also* Clinical application
    of exercise
Exercise programs. *See* Clinical application of exercise
Exercise testing. *See also* Screening for exercise therapy
  with complications of Type I diabetes, 155, 158, 159
  with Type II diabetes in general, 171, 173

F
Faber, O., 44-45
Fat metabolism, in exercise response with Type I diabetes, 42. *See also* Adipose
    tissue, metabolism in
Felig, P., 38, 40, 43, 98
Ferrannini, E., 44-45
Finkelstein, J.A., 96
Flexibility exercises. *See* Stretching exercises
Fluid replacement with exercise therapy, 152, 161
Follow-up for exercise therapy, with Type I diabetes, 161-162
Foot injury, avoiding, 156
Footwear for exercise, 156, 160-161, 179-180
Free fatty acids (FFA) in exercise response
  with Type I diabetes, 42, 45, 53
  with Type II diabetes, 95, 97, 100
  without diabetes, 86, 87
Free insulin levels, in exercise response with Type I diabetes, 48, 49
Freinkel, N., 38
Frequency of training, 178
Frid, A., 150
Friedman, J.E., 96
Fuller, S., 41-42
Furler, S.M., 94

G
Garretto, L., 88
Gestational diabetes, 182
Ginsberg-Fellner, F., 130
Glucagon and exercise response
  with Type I diabetes, 35, 36, 37, 48, 49, 53
  with Type II diabetes, 97
  without diabetes, 87, 91
Gluconeogenesis, 12, 36, 41, 87, 92
Glucose clamp technique, 67
Glucose levels. *See also* Glycemic control; Hyperglycemia; Hypoglycemia
  in exercise response

Glucose levels (*continued*)
    with Type I diabetes, 35-37, 44, 45, 48-53
    with Type II diabetes, 93-101
    without diabetes, 88
  monitoring of, with exercise programs, 147, 179
  in training adaptations
    with Type I diabetes, 61-66
    with Type II diabetes, 117, 118-120, 121, 129, 130, 181-182
Glucose production/uptake
  complications of diabetes and, 16
  in exercise response
    with Type I diabetes, 35-42, 43, 45
    with Type II diabetes, 92-93
    without diabetes, 86, 88, 89-92
  in training adaptations
    with Type I diabetes, 67-71
    with Type II diabetes, 121, 122, 123
    without diabetes, 116
  with Type II diabetes in general, 11-12
Glucose tolerance, oral, in training adaptations with Type II diabetes, 119, 120, 122
Glucose transport
  in exercise response
    with Type I diabetes, 39-40
    with Type II diabetes, 92-93, 96, 97, 100
    without diabetes, 89, 92
  in training adaptations
    with Type I diabetes, 70-71
    with Type II diabetes, 123, 126, 127
Glycemic control. *See also* Glucose levels; Insulin treatment
  in adaptation to training
    with Type I diabetes, 61-66
    with Type II diabetes, 118-120, 121, 129, 130
  in clinical applications
    with Type I diabetes, 146-152, 161
    with Type II diabetes, 178-179
  in exercise response with Type II diabetes, 92-101
Glycemic excursions, 46
Glycemic state/response, with Type I diabetes, 35, 36, 44. *See also* Glucose levels;
    Glucose production/uptake; Glycemic control; Hyperglycemia; Hypoglycemia
Glycogen
  exercise response and
    with Type I diabetes, 42, 43
    with Type II diabetes, 98
    without diabetes, 86, 87, 88
  replacing reserves following exercise therapy, 148
  training adaptations and
    with Type I diabetes, 72-74
    without diabetes, 116
Glycogenolysis, 12, 36, 43, 87, 92
Glycolytic glucose utilization, in exercise response, 38
Glycosylated hemoglobin (hemoglobin A_{1c}), 3-4, 62, 65, 119, 130, 181
Goodman, M.N., 88
Goodyear, L.J., 70
Gordon, Neil, 162

Gorski, J., 100
Graham, T., 72
Greenfield, M.S., 13
Greenlee, G., 158
Gries, F.A., 48
Growth hormone
    in exercise response, 48, 49, 53
    with retinopathy, 157
Gunnarsson, R., 46-48, 77

H

Hagenfeldt, L., 38, 40
Hagg, S., 38
Hanna, A.K., 95
HbA$_{1c}$ (glycosylated hemoglobin), 3-4, 62, 65, 119, 130, 181
HDL. *See* High-density lipoprotein (HDL) levels
Heart rate, for monitoring exercise, 175-177
Heath, G.W., 181-182
Hedig, L., 43
Hemoglobin A$_{1c}$, 3-4, 62, 65, 119, 130, 181
Hepatic insulin resistance, 10, 12
High-density lipoprotein (HDL) levels
    exercise in general and, 20
    in training adaptations
        with Type I diabetes, 75, 77
        with Type II diabetes, 128, 129, 181
        with Type I diabetes in general, 13-14, 181
        with Type II diabetes in general, 13, 181
Hirshman, M.F., 70
Histocompatibility antigens, 2-3
Hoeldtke, R.D., 154
Holloszy, J.O., 70, 93, 120, 121
Holly, R.G., 128-129
Honeymoon phase, 3
Hormones, in exercise response with Type II diabetes, 96-97
Horton, E.S., 43, 70, 97-98, 100, 101
Houmard, J.A., 71
Houston, M., 72
Hubinger, A., 48
Huh, K.B., 119
Human insulin, guidelines for use with exercise therapy, 150
Hyde, R.T., 78
Hydration with exercise therapy, 152, 161
Hyperglycemia
    exercise precautions with, 147
    in exercise response
        with Type I diabetes, 37, 38, 41, 46
        with Type II diabetes, 96
        without diabetes, 90-91
    training adaptations with Type II diabetes and, 120
Hypertension
    complications of diabetes and, 16
    effect of exercise on, 20
    in exercise response with Type II diabetes, 103

Hypertension (*continued*)
  exercise therapy with, 146
Hypoglycemia
  in exercise response
    with Type I diabetes, 36, 37, 44, 45, 46, 53
    with Type II diabetes, 97
    without diabetes, 91
  guidelines for avoiding
    with complications of Type I diabetes, 155
    with Type I diabetes in general, 144, 147, 148, 150-151, 152
    with Type II diabetes in general, 179
  in training adaptations with Type II diabetes, 122
Hypotension, 154

I

Injection site, 44-45, 150-151, 178
Injury prevention. *See* Precautions for exercise
Insulin. *See also* Insulin binding; Insulin in exercise response; Insulin levels; Insulin
    resistance; Insulin secretion; Insulin sensitivity; Insulin treatment
  basic function of, 35
  thermic effects of, 101
Insulin binding
  with Type I diabetes, 71
  with Type II diabetes, 93, 98, 100, 126
  without diabetes, 88
Insulin clamp technique, 101
Insulin dependent diabetes mellitus (IDDM). *See* Type I diabetes (insulin depen-
    dent diabetes mellitus, IDDM)
Insulin in exercise response
  blood glucose levels and, 36-37, 38-40, 43, 45, 89, 91, 96-97, 100, 101
  overview of, 18
  with Type I diabetes
    blood glucose and, 36-37, 38-40, 43, 45
    exercise intensity/duration and, 48-53
    injection site and, 44-45
    mode of insulin treatment and, 46-48
    pharmacokinetics of insulin and, 45
  with Type II diabetes, 96-97, 100, 101
  without diabetes, 89, 91
Insulin levels
  in exercise response
    with Type II diabetes, 94-95, 97
    without diabetes, 87, 88
  exercise therapy and, 148, 178
  training adaptations with Type II diabetes and, 119, 122
Insulin resistance
  complications of diabetes and, 16
  in exercise response
    with Type I diabetes, 39, 43
    with Type II diabetes, 92-93, 95-96
    without diabetes, 88
  training adapatations
    with Type II diabetes, 121
    without diabetes, 116, 117
  with Type II diabetes in general, 8, 10, 11

Insulin secretion
  abnormal, in general, 8-9
  complications of diabetes and, 16
  in exercise response, 87, 95
  normal (without diabetes), 7, 87
  with Type II diabetes
    in exercise response, 95
    in training adaptations, 119, 120-121, 122-123
Insulin sensitivity
  in exercise response
    with Type I diabetes, 42-43
    with Type II diabetes, 93, 98, 100-101
    without diabetes, 88-89
  in training adaptations
    with Type I diabetes, 66-71, 72
    with Type II diabetes, 117, 120, 121-123, 124-125, 126
    without diabetes, 66-71, 72
Insulin treatment
  activity characteristics and, 149
  exercise response with Type I diabetes and, 44-48
  with exercise therapy
    with Type I diabetes, 148-152
    with Type II diabetes, 178-179
  injection site and, 44-45, 150-151, 178
  mode of, 46-48, 151-152
Intensity of exercise
  clinical applications
    with complications of Type I diabetes, 154, 155, 160
    with Type II diabetes, 170, 173-174, 175-177
  exercise response and
    with Type I diabetes, 48-53
    with Type II diabetes, 88
    without diabetes, 86, 88, 89
  methods for monitoring, 175-177
Intermediate-acting insulin, 148-149
Intracellular membrane (IM), 39
Intramuscular injection, and exercise therapy, 150
Ischemia, 102-103
Ismail, A.H., 128
Ivy, J.L., 126

J
Jacobsen, U.K., 65, 67, 71
James, D.E., 70, 89
Jenkins, A.B., 94
Jorgensen, F.S., 65, 67, 71
Joslin Clinic, 77
Jovanovic-Peterson, L., 182
Juvenile-onset diabetes. *See* Type I diabetes (insulin-dependent diabetes mellitus, IDDM)

K
Karnielli, E., 100
Kawamori, R., 45
Kelly, D., 44

Kemmer, F.W., 44, 45
Kendrick, J.S., 181-182
Ketoacidosis, 3
Ketones, 42
Ketosis, 38
Khachadurian, A.K., 53, 129, 180-181
Kiens, B., 72, 75
Kim, H.C., 129
Kjaer, M., 96
Klip, A., 39, 89
Koivisto, V.A., 93-94, 98, 100
Krokiweski, M., 72, 75
Krotkiewski, M., 100, 122
Krzentowski, P., 42

L

Laitinen, J., 119
Lampman, Richard M., 119, 121, 127, 181
Landt, K.W., 62, 67
Länsimies, E., 119
LaPorte, R.E., 77
Lattimore, L., 128-129
LDL. *See* Low-density lipoprotein (LDL) levels
Left ventricular function
    clinincal application guidelines and, 161
    in exercise response with Type II diabetes, 102
Lehmann, E., 48
Leiter, L.A., 95
Lemon, P.W., 96
Leonard, B.E., 181-182
Levinson, G.E., 38
Life expectancy, 15, 77-78
Lilia, B., 154, 157
Linde, B., 44-45, 150
Linde, R., 150
Lipid levels
    abnormalities in, 12-14
    complications of diabetes and, 16
    exercise in general and, 20
    exercise response with Type II diabetes and, 103
    in training adaptations
        with Type I diabetes, 75-77
        with Type II diabetes, 117, 128, 129, 130
    with Type I diabetes in general, 12, 13-14
    with Type II diabetes in general, 12-13, 14
Lipoprotein levels. *See also* High-density lipoprotein (HDL) levels
    abnormalities in, 12-14
    exercise in general and, 20
    of low-density lipoprotein (LDL), 20, 75, 77, 129
    in training adaptations
        with Type I diabetes, 72, 75-77
        with Type II diabetes, 129
    with Type I diabetes in general, 12, 13-14, 181
    with Type II diabetes in general, 12-13, 14, 181

of very-low-density lipoprotein (VLDL), 13, 14
Lithell, H., 72, 75
Long-acting insulin, 149, 152
Low-density lipoprotein (LDL) levels, 20, 75, 77, 129

M
Macrovascular complications
   description of, 14
   exercise response with Type II diabetes and, 103
   training adaptatation with Type I diabetes and, 77
Maehlum, S., 92
Maladjustment, psychosocial, 15
Manhem, P., 154
Mann, J.I., 14
Marliss, E.B., 46, 95
Maturity-onset diabetes. *See* Type II diabetes (non-insulin dependent diabetes
      mellitus, NIDDM)
Maximal heart rate, 175-177
Maximal oxygen comsumption (VO₂max), in training adaptations with Type II
      diabetes, 127-128, 181
McDermott, J.C., 116
Megeney, L.A., 126
Metabolic control. *See* Glucose levels; Glycemic control
Metabolism in muscles. *See* Skeletal muscle metabolism, training adaptations in
Microvascular complications
   description of, 14
   exercise response with Type II diabetes and, 103
Mikines, K.J., 88
Minuk, H.L., 95, 118
Mode of exercise, with Type II diabetes, 174. *See also* Aerobic exercise; Resistance
      (strength) training; Stretching exercises
Mode of insulin treatment, 46-48
Mogensen, C.E., 159
Mondon, C.E., 70
Monitoring, in exercise programs
   of glucose levels, 147, 179
   of heart rate/exercise intensity, 175-177
Monocytes, insulin binding to, 71, 98, 100, 126
Moy, C.S., 77-78
Muscle capillarization in training adaptations
   with Type I diabetes, 75
   with Type II diabetes, 123, 126
   without diabetes, 123
Muscle enzymes
   in exercise response with Type II diabetes, 97
   in training adaptations with Type I diabetes, 72, 73
Muscle metabolism. *See* Skeletal muscle metabolism, training adaptations in
Mustonen, J.N., 102

N
Naka, M., 102-103
National Health and Nutrition Examination Survey (NHANES), 4
Nephropathy
   description of, 14, 159-160
   exercise therapy with Type I diabetes and, 146, 160-161

Neuropathy
    description of, 14, 153-154, 155-156
    exercise therapy for, with Type I diabetes, 154-157
Non-insulin dependent diabetes mellitus (NIDDM). *See* Type II diabetes (non-insulin dependent diabetes mellitus, NIDDM)
Noradrenaline response, 154
Norepinephrine in exercise response
    with Type I diabetes, 35, 49, 53
    with Type II diabetes, 95, 97
Nygaard, E., 72

O

Obesity. *See also* Weight loss
    complications of diabetes and, 16
    exercise benefits for, 20
    glucose production/uptake and, 11-12
    insulin secretion with, 9
    with Type II diabetes
        exercise response and, 94-96, 98, 100
        training adaptations and, 119, 126-127, 129-130
Oral glucose tolerance, in training adaptations with Type II diabetes, 119, 120, 122
Osteoporosis, 20
Ostman, J., 150

P

Paffenbarger, R.S., Jr., 78
Painter, P., 160
Pandolfi, M., 157
Parikh, S., 45
Pedersen, O., 65, 67, 71
Pederson, O., 43
Peripheral insulin resistance, 10
Peripheral neuropathy, 146, 155-157
Peripheral vascular disease, 15, 20
Peterson, C.M., 182
Pharmacokinetics of insulin, 45
Physician's role in program design, 141, 144
Piper, R.C., 89
Ploug, T., 70
Postabsorptive state, 46
Postexercise recovery
    with Type II diabetes, 95, 97-98, 99, 101
    without diabetes, 91-92, 116
Postprandial exercise, 45. *See also* Dietary intake
Poussier, P., 46
Powell, K.E., 181-182
Precautions for exercise
    with Type I diabetes
        in general, 144, 145-147
        with nephropathy, 161
        with neuropathy, 155, 156-157, 161-162
        with retinopathy, 158-159
    with Type II diabetes, 178, 179
Pregnancy, 182

Prescription of exercise with Type II diabetes, 173-178. *See also* Clinical application of exercise
Pritikin, N., 128-129
Progression of effort, 177-178
Proteinuria, 159
Psychosocial maladjustment, 15
Pulse rate, for monitoring exercise, 175-177
Pyke, D.A., 8
Pyruvate dehydrogenase activity, 42

R

Recovery. *See* Postexercise recovery
Reitman, J.S., 118, 120
Renal disease risk level, 15. *See also* Nephropathy
Resistance (strength) training
   with nephropathy, 160, 161
   physiological/metabolic adaptations to, 18
   with retinopathy, 158
   with Type I diabetes, 65, 158
Response to acute exercise
   normal (without diabetes), 17, 86-92
   with Type I diabetes
      diet and, 44, 46, 48
      elevated insulin levels and, 45-46
      glucose production/utilization and, 35-42, 43, 45
      insulin binding, 71
      insulin injection site and, 44-45
      insulin sensitivity and, 42-43
      insulin treatment modality and, 46-48
      intensity/duration and, 48-53
   with Type II diabetes
      blood glucose control, 92-101
      cardiovascular, 101-104
      diet and, 95
      insulin sensitivity and, 93, 98, 100-101
      intensity and, 88
Retinopathy
   description of, 14, 157-158
   exercise response with Type II diabetes and, 102, 103
   exercise therapy with Type I diabetes and, 146, 158-159
Richter, E.A., 88
Ridderskamp, I., 48
Risks of exercise. *See also* Precautions for exercise
   with Type I diabetes
      in general, 144-147
      with neuropathy, 154-155, 156, 160
      with retinopathy, 158
   with Type II diabetes, 170, 172, 180
Rodnick, K.J., 70, 89
Romanelli, G., 104
Rönnemaa, T., 119
Rossner, S., 77
Rowland, T.W., 62
Ruderman, N., 129

Ruderman, N.B., 38, 88
Ruderman, N.D., 180-181

S
Safety. *See* Precautions for exercise; Risks of exercise
Saltin, B., 72, 75
Sanders, C.A., 38
Sarcolemma, 40, 70
Schneider, S.H., 53, 119, 129, 180-181
Schriffrin, A., 45
Schteingart, D.E., 119
Screening for exercise therapy. *See also* Exercise testing
    with Type I diabetes, 140-141, 155
    with Type II diabetes, 169-170, 171-172, 173
Scrimgeour, A., 41-42
Segal, K.R., 122, 130
Shamoon, H., 36
Shapiro, Y., 100
Shilo, S., 36
Shoes for exercise, 156, 160-161, 179-180
Short-acting insulin, 149-150, 152
Siitonen, O., 119
Silent myocardial ischemia, 102-103
Skeletal muscle metabolism, training adaptations in
    with Type I diabetes, 72-75
    with Type II diabetes, 118, 123, 126-127
Slot, J.W., 89
Soman, V.R., 98
Somatostatin, 36
Sotsky, M., 36
Special needs patients, 182. *See also* Complications of diabetes
Strength training. *See* Resistance (strength) training
Stretching exercises
    with neuropathy with Type I diabetes, 156
    with Type II diabetes, 174-175
Stroke, cerebral, 15
Sundvist, G., 154, 157

T
Tajima, N., 77
Takahashi, N., 102
Tan, M.H., 43, 71, 116
Timing of insulin treatment, 151-152
Torgan, C.E., 126
Training. *See* Adaptation to training; Clinical application of exercise
Treatment for diabetes, medical, 16-17. *See also* Clinical application of exercise;
    Insulin treatment
Triglyceride levels
    exercise in general and, 20
    in training adaptations
        with Type I diabetes, 75, 77
        with Type II diabetes, 129, 181
    with Type I diabetes in general, 14, 181
    with Type II diabetes in general, 13, 14, 181
Trovati, M., 46, 121

Type I diabetes (insulin dependent diabetes mellitus, IDDM). *See also* Adaptation to training, with Type I diabetes; Clinical application of exercise, with Type I diabetes; Response to acute exercise, with Type I diabetes
  characteristics of, overview, 1-4, 6
  complications of, overview, 3, 14-16
  diet with, 44, 46, 48, 147-148, 152
  exercise benefits with, 144-147, 152, 160
  lipid/lipoprotein abnormalities with, 12, 13-14
  medical treatment of, 16
Type IB diabetes, 3
Type II diabetes (non-insulin dependent diabetes mellitus, NIDDM). *See also* Adaptation to training, with Type II diabetes; Clinical application of exercise, with Type II diabetes; Response to acute exercise, with Type II diabetes
  abnormalities with, overview, 8-12, 14
  characteristics of, overview, 4-7
  complications of, overview, 5, 14-16
  diet with, 95, 119, 121, 128-130, 170
  exercise benefits with, 169-170, 171
  exercise for prevention of, 19
  medical treatment of, 16-17

U
Uusitupa, M., 119

V
Valsalva maneuver, 158, 160
Valyou, P.M., 70
Vanninen, E., 119
Ventricular function. *See* Left ventricular function
Verity, L.S., 128
Very-low-density lipoprotein (VLDL), 13, 14
Vittinghus, K., 159
Vitug, A., 53
VO$_2$max, in training adaptations with Type II diabetes, 127-128, 181
Vranic, M., 45, 95

W
Wahren, J., 38, 40, 41, 72, 77
Wallberg-Henriksson, H., 46-48, 65, 67, 72, 75, 77, 93, 127
Warm-up and cool-down, 174-175, 178
Wasserman, D.H., 36
Weight lifting. *See* Resistance (strength) training
Weight loss, in training adaptations with Type II diabetes, 129-130. *See also* Obesity
Wilson, R.H., 181-182
Wing, A.L., 78

Y
Yale, J.F., 95
Yki-jarvinen, H., 65, 67, 100

Z
Zander, E., 45
Zinman, B., 44, 45, 46, 65, 95
Zuniga-Guajardo, S., 44
Zuni Indians, 181-182

About the Authors

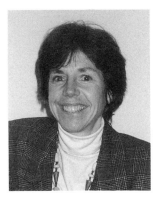

Barbara Campaigne

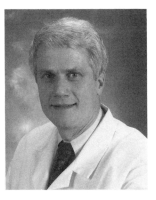

Richard Lampman

Barbara N. Campaigne, PhD, is the director of research development at the American College of Sports Medicine (ACSM). Since 1979 she has extensively researched the effects of exercise on diabetes in the United States and Sweden. She was a visiting scholar at the world-renowned Karolinska Institute in Stockholm during 1986 and received a research grant from the Swedish Diabetes Association. Dr. Campaigne previously served as a research scientist in the division of cardiology at Children's Hospital in Cincinnati, Ohio.

Dr. Campaigne chaired the 1988 Symposium on Diabetes and Exercise conducted by ACSM. In 1987 she was named Diabetes Educator of the Year by the Ohio affiliate of the American Diabetes Association, of which she is a member. Dr. Campaigne is also a member and fellow of ACSM and a member of the International Diabetic Athletes Association.

Richard M. Lampman, PhD, is the director of research in the Department of General Surgery at Catherine McAuley Health System, Ann Arbor, Michigan. He also serves as research director in the peripheral vascular laboratory at St. Joseph Mercy Hospital in Ann Arbor. Dr. Lampman previously served as a research scientist in the division of cardiology at the University of Michigan Medical Center, Ann Arbor. He is currently an adjunct associate professor at the University of Michigan at Ann Arbor.

Dr. Lampman is an ACSM fellow and a consultant to the Department of Health and Human Services in educational programs for health professionals caring for Native Americans with Type II diabetes. He also serves as a grant reviewer for the National Institutes of Health and the National Heart, Lung, and Blood Institute. Dr. Lampman is a frequent contributor to scientific journals, writing on cardiology and endocrinology.